BY THE NUMBERS

A Guide to Buying and Running Your Dental Practice

Addison Killeen, DDS

Forward by Mark Costes, DDS

2018 Paperback Edition

© 2017, 2018 Addison Killeen, DDS

All rights reserved.

Published in the United States by CreateSpace Independent Publishing Platform, an imprint of Amazon.

Library of Congress Cataloging-in-Publication Data
Killeen, Addison.

By the Numbers: A Guide to Buying and Running Your Dental Practice / by Addison Killeen, DDS

ISBN-13:978-1973856801 - ISBN-10: 1973856808
1. Dentistry 2. Dental Office Practice

Acknowledgements

There are tons of people whom I'd like to thank for their help with this book. First and foremost are my parents. Their love and support through my childhood created a love of learning and the security to try new things. I am especially thankful for my mother as an editor of my ideas and the original numbers guru. Even today, I can call her with an Excel issue and she will help me through it! My father taught me the value of hard work and being a good family man. His work ethic and integrity are second to none. Also to my brothers, who helped me form these ideas over coffee and bike rides- sorry the inevitable boring conversation. I'd also like to thank all the team members at all the locations of Williamsburg Dental - who have grown the practice and helped refine the ideas presented in this book.

Thanks to Kevin Rossen of Divergent Dental for all the late night and early morning texts and emails. He helped me to clarify my ideas and present these ideas with the data to back them. His mission to bring good data to the industry aligns closely with my passion of running a dental practice with good data. I'm also thankful for Michael Lomotan who helped clarify some of the good data, and always bringing a positive spirit to life.

I would like to thank my wife Rachel most of all, for being patient with all my neurotic tendencies. From waking up way too early in the morning, to talking about dentistry all times of the day and night, your support and love is unbelievable. I'm looking forward to our boys growing up knowing more than they should about dentistry!

By the Numbers

A Guide to Buying and Running Your Dental Practice

Foreword by Dr. Mark Costes
Founder of Dental Success Institute

1. How to use this book
   a. What do I know?   11
   b. How to read this book   13

2. Starting (or Buying) a Dental Office   15
   a. Valuation   16
      i. EBITDA   17
      ii. Other Factors   23
      iii. Allocation of Assets   25
      iv. Accounts Receivable   29
   b. Financing   33
      i. Working Capital   35
      ii. Pro Forma Statement   36
      iii. Personal Financial Statement   39
   c. Startup Documents & Plan   40
   d. Legal Issues and Taxes   47
      i. Tax Strategy   49

3. Watching the Numbers   57
   a. Leading Indicators   61
      i. Weekly   63
      ii. Monthly   74
   b. Key Production Indicators   84
   c. Numbers to Track Intermittently   101

4. Final Notes   107

Foreword

Dr. Mark Costes

Growing up as child with attention and learning challenges, dentistry was never on my radar early in life. That all changed in my junior year of high school when, in my very first varsity baseball game, I collided at full speed, face-first into the left field fence. And in that split second, the course of my life was altered forever.

The accident had left me with several avulsed and fractured teeth as well as a broken jaw. The fourteen months that followed were spent in the offices of multiple dentists and dental specialists. These professionals worked together in a coordinated effort to correct the traumatic injuries to my mouth, face and jaw.

On the other side of it, I had a brand new smile with minimal scarring, and a profound respect for the profession of dentistry. I grew to admire those who dedicated their lives to developing this unique skill set- which I now viewed as a combination of medicine, artistry and technical precision.

My new course was set. I was going to be a dentist. The problem was, although I now had a clear vision and desire, my challenges with reading and comprehension left me with test scores and a GPA that were average not exceptional.

My experience with the dental school application process was long and tedious. During undergrad, I had served in leadership positions in my national fraternity and had logged hundreds of hours volunteering in dental offices and for community-based non-profits. In my essay, I told the story of how a group of dental professionals restored my smile and inspired me to be able to do the same one day... but would the non-academic elements of my background be enough to overcome the otherwise average nature of my application?

For years, the answer to this question remained a definitive "no." Over a three-year period of time, I submitted 21 applications; I was rejected 20 times and received a single acceptance.

Looking back, although this was one of the most difficult periods of my life, both emotionally and financially, it was also the most formative. During this period of time, I applied and was accepted to an Executive MBA program at the University of San Diego. I was also able to flex my entrepreneurial muscle when I purchased my first business, a catering truck franchise.

While the MBA curriculum exposed me to theory and case studies, running my own business provided me with a *real* education. It was baptism by fire. Figure it out or close up shop. Learn how to profit or perish. This business gave me real world experience in human resources, marketing, customer service, and the ability to read financial reports.

Within months, the business went from fledgling upstart to one of the best in the fleet -- a thriving and profitable business. But more importantly, the experience helped me to develop the ability to analyze and interpret business analytics.

In retrospect, it was these years of struggle and rejection that ended up being the foundation of all of my future business endeavors. In the years since what I now call, my "gap" years, I've owned and operated several successful businesses- including 14 dental offices.

I read the manuscript of ***By the Numbers*** from cover to cover on a non-stop flight from Phoenix to Orlando with pen and highlighter in hand and didn't put it down once. Addison presents the numbers behind the successful operation of a dental practice in a clear succinct and masterful way.

From novice to advanced, and for anyone who owns or is considering owning a single or multiple dental offices, this is a must read. Dr. Killeen de-mystifies such topics as Practice Valuation, EBITDA, KPI's and Leading Indicators with no-nonsense language and real-world examples.

I'm honored to have been tasked with writing the foreword to this book, a book that I am confident will change the lives and improve the businesses of practice owners in this generation and many to come.

Committed to your Success,

Mark Costes, DDS

Founder, Dental Success Institute
Founder, Horizon Schools of Dental Assisting
Author of the #1 International Bestselling Book, *Pillars of Dental Success*
Host, *The Dentalpreneur Podcast*

What do I know?

There are many books out there discussing how to run your dental practice. There are also many consultants out there who will gladly come help you run your office for a briefcase filled with cash. I'm not here to come into your office and turn you into someone that you wouldn't like looking at in the mirror. My only purpose in this book is to share knowledge that will help you run your business better. From one dentist to another, I want every dental office to be run well and efficiently. This book is the culmination of proof that when you run your business better, you can have a less stressful life and enjoy financial success!

My central mantra in bringing this information to you is that *information is power.* You don't know what you haven't measured. How do you know what bonding agent to use unless someone has studied it and looked at its bond strengths? How do you know what impression material to use unless someone measures the elasticity and accuracy? Information is what leads us to improving all aspects of our dentistry. Sadly, **many dentists often poor business decisions** make, or just average ones, based on misinformation and 'gut feelings' that are not correct. We often see things like an empty schedule or a new insurance plan on the market and make poor decisions based on this new information.

My experience comes from two sources. I was lucky enough at a young age to have a mentor who ran a conglomerate of businesses in different industries. This man was a visionary, and he built up numerous businesses on different models. From designing machines for the Department of Defense, to running restaurants and a brewery, he always looked at the numbers. As a young kid following him around, I was able to gain a feeling for how the business world works. In the restaurant industry, almost 80% of restaurants will close before their 5th anniversary. The margins on the food and hospitality industry are razor thin. They are happy to get 3% profit margin over the course of a year. In any well-run restaurant, they know the exact cost of the salmon filet, the butter on top, and the green beans beside it. Are you ordering the special today? That's because they got a good deal on a case of chicken parmesan ingredients, and those ingredients have a better profitability than other menu items. It's ALL about the numbers in a restaurant. When you operate on a very thin profit margin, every percentage point counts.

Another thing I learned from my work experience is that **you don't need an MBA to run your business**. The CEO I worked for always said, "I don't have a PhD in finance, but I've taken all the classes." This was absolutely true, as he had sat through many hours of coursework to become intensely knowledgeable about how to run his businesses.

We dentists don't need to learn about high corporate finance to be able to run our shops in the best way. We don't need to learn about *cross-functional and cross-firm technological integration*. All we need to do is know our data and use that to make informed and smart business decisions. We went to 8 years or more of higher education, so we are all capable of executing at the highest levels.

With any endeavor, there will be mistakes. I've made a ton, and I continue to everyday. The key is to move on, get better, and learn from the mistakes. This book will help you learn the systems that will enable you to hopefully avoid a few mistakes, increase your profitability, and have more fun doing dentistry!

How to Use this Book:

So you picked up this book because you're thinking about owning your own shop, or running your practice better. You will not be disappointed! Dentistry is one of the best careers out there, as proven by US News & World Report constantly ranking General Dentists and Orthodontists in the top 3 year after year. If you are reading this book, you are in the driver's seat for a great career!

Now, this book is not to be read on a quiet beach sometime when you are relaxing. This book is all about running your business better. To that end, this is more of a workbook than something to be read front to back. Read each chapter at a point in time when it is useful, and then put it back on your bookshelf. At some point, many of these chapters will apply to your business. Some you may never touch.

If you are reading this book, you are already showing that you're driven to be successful. Here are some of the 'must-read' books from Dr. Mark Costes and the Dental Success Institute:
- The 4 Disciplines of Execution by Sean Covey and others
- Extreme Ownership – Jocko Willink and Leif Babin
- The E-Myth Revisited by Michael Gerber
- The Ultimate Sales Machine by Chet Holmes
- The Obstacle is the Way by Ryan Holiday

If you're itching to be an owner, run the shop, and be successful, then you need to read this and then keep going further. Go to more Continuing Education sessions, find friends who are also running their shops, and share with older dentists who have already been successful. There are many CE opportunities around that discuss business acumen. There are also many resources that are absolutely free, like Podcasts and Blogs from the leading thinkers in the industry. This book is not intended to replace every learning opportunity out there. If it were, it would be as thick as a dictionary or periodontics textbook. This book is meant to kick-start your learning and help you become as successful as possible. This book is also meant to teach the most useful and powerful tools to get you to financial success and business success.

As with almost everything these days, there needs to be a disclaimer about the legal, accounting and tax advice in this book. I am not an accountant, and this should not be considered tax advice. I am not a lawyer and this should not be considered legal advice. You should seek appropriate counsel for your own situation. And please note, this is directed toward readers in the United States. If you are conducting business outside of the United States, I highly encourage you to find and understand your legal obligations in your country.

Since we are through with that, let's jump into the first issue that most dentists face as they approach practice ownership- practice valuation.

Starting (or Buying) a dental office

"Whatever the mind can conceive and believe, the mind can achieve." -- Napoleon Hill

So you just graduated, and you're thinking, "What do I do now?" The world of dentistry has endless possibilities for you. There's a corporate practice in Colorado where you can ski on the weekends or on your days off. There's a small town practice in Wyoming where you can live on the lake and be the central figure in town. You could buy an office in Manhattan and have a view overlooking New York City!

When assessing any opportunity, there are hundreds of things to be thinking about. Will the selling doctor stay working for you? Will the staff of the selling doctor stay with the company? If purchasing an existing dental practice is the way to go right now, read this valuation chapter and use the tools to come to an appropriate purchase price.

Valuation & Financing

When you start looking to buy an office, the first two questions you will ask is, "How much does it cost, and how will I pay for it?" When it comes to the question of cost, it often comes with a perceived value from the seller. Knowing a good valuation approach is key. There are a few methods out there, but there is one that almost every accountant will understand. After answering the first question, then we will cover how to go to a bank/institution to ask to borrow the money for it.

Valuation

There are a couple of reliable methods that are used to determine the value of a dental practice if you will be the sole practitioner of the entity. Some selling doctors think it is a percentage of historical revenues, or some other measure similar to this. However, we should look at the bigger picture, and the important data. Rather than using methods created in a cottage dental practice industry, we need to treat this like a business. When looking at a practice, some methods leave many aspects out. Of course there are many other ways to say how much it is worth, but in the end it comes down to only the price at which the seller and buyer agree. Value equals sales price. So how do we get to that point?

EBITDA

EBITDA stands for 'earnings before interest, taxes, depreciation, and amortization'. Basically, EBITDA is the cash earnings of the business without all the tax implications, which really only happen after you make money. When you start any valuation, it is always good to get the prior 3 years tax returns from the seller's business. Three years gives a decent picture of the average collections of the business, and since it is reported to the IRS, usually you can trust that it is true. Of course some people rob the IRS of due taxes, but hopefully that's not the person selling to you! The other more detailed way to get these numbers is to get the actual Profit and Loss statements from the seller or their accountant. The P&L as we call it, will give you a proper look at all the collections and small expense categories that can be lost on the IRS forms. These P&L statements will help you understand what cost categories may be high or low based on what kind of work the prior owner is doing. It may even give you an idea of ways to improve the profitability of the practice once you take ownership.

> Go to Addisonkilleen.com to download the EBITDA spreadsheet to do all these calculations automatically.

Step 1: Normalize
Once you have 3 years of tax returns or P&L statements, then you need to normalize each year. Often dentists will run many costs through the business that may, shall we say, not be *completely* business related. This may include the doctor's entire family cell phone bill, their home internet (for home office use of course), their car, and occasionally their boat- because staff team building happens on that boat.

> Note: Concerning the running of expenses through your business: Many expenses can be run through your business. Meals with people when you meet them on business related topics are quite common. Vehicle expenses are another common one. One accountant once told me, "Pigs get fat, hogs get slaughtered. Basically, you want to maximize expenses that are business related, but don't push the limit. Don't be going 65mph in a 55 mph zone." To this rule: vehicle expenses should be kept at a moderate level. One way that the IRS sees as favorable is to lease a car, and have the company pay the lease costs. The cost of taxes, title, licensing, gas, and repairs should be paid for through your personal account.

The best way to normalize the income is to copy the most recent P&L into a spreadsheet. In column A, list the P&L categories. In column B, put the costs from the dental practice as it is currently being run. In column C, reduce any costs to what they would actually be once you remove all the 'perks' of being the dentist owner. These costs include travel, CE, and other items that aren't critical to the running of the business. Sometimes they also include donations, or advertising expenses that are really just set up as donations. For example, perhaps the previous dentist sponsored his child's baseball team, but will that continue? They gave $2,000 to the *Save the Beetles* campaign, but is this expense critical to the business success? After removing those costs, all those perks should be added into the profitability of the practice. See the simple example below in Table 1.1. Column D is then the 'normalized' P&L from the practice, and this column will give you the most accurate 'profit' from the practice.

The current dentist is taking home $104,360 as 'profit' from his business. After taking out the car, donations, and other expenses that the new dentist will not incur, then the profit jumps to $123,000. This new 'normalized profit' is the first starting number for the next calculation.

Important to this exercise is assigning salary levels for the owner or associate dentists. This can be something from $80,000 to $180,000. This impacts taxes for the seller as they take income, but also impacts valuation. For a practice, try to use a calculation that is typical for an associate or senior dentist working in the area. If the practice is producing $600,000, it is not realistic to pay the dentist $60,000, or 10%. First and foremost, if the IRS notices this, they will probably perform an audit and back taxes might be owed. Secondly, you will never get a dentist to come in and do dentistry and take home only 10% of collections. Finding associates is hard, and finding ones that will work for 10% is impossible. In this scenario, and in general, you should make the dentist's salary as much as 25% of collections. However, if your collections are going over $600,000, you could reasonably cap the salary at $150,000.

Table 1.1	2017 P&L	Normalized	New P&L
Income	600,000		600,000
Staff costs	180,000		180,000
Dentist Salary	150,000		150,000
Supplies	36,000		36,000
Lab Fees	48,000		48,000
Vehicle	7,640	-7640	0
Office Costs	17,800		17,800
Rent	24,700		24,700
Donations	2,000	-2000	0
Advertising	15,000		15,000
Travel and CE	9,000	-9000	0
Other	5,500		5,500
Profit	$104,360		Normalized: $123,000

> Note: Watch for a selling dentist to try to normalize the profit as high as possible. It is in their interest to get that profit number up-thereby increasing the value of the practice. At this point all normalization becomes a negotiation. Hopefully all parties in the transaction realize true business expenses, so there can be a fairly easy agreement on the actual profit level of the practice.

Step 2: Once you perform this 'normalization' exercise for each of the previous 3 years, then you can perform the EBIDTA calculation. Table 1.2 shows the calculation.

Table 1.2			Most Recent Year
	2014	2015	2016
EBIDTA	$113,000	$117,500	$123,000
Weighted Multiple	1	2	3
	$113,000	$235,000	$369,000
Total	$717,000		
Multiple	6		
Total divided by Multiple =	$119,500	Average Weighted EBITDA	

As you can see, the previous 2 years weren't as profitable as the most recent. It is prudent to give more weight to the most recent year, because hopefully the new dentist can match that production and income. Previous years have less weight because of different factors including different rents, costs, and the overall economy.

After multiplying the EBITDA by the weight, you then add all the totals together for a large sum. In this scenario, it is $717,000. Since you multiplied all the previous numbers by 1, 2 and 3, then you add those together for a total of 6. Then divide $717,000 by 6 to get your annualized average weighted EBITDA.

> Hint: If you were to look at 4 years of returns, you would take the weights of 1, 2, 3, and 4, and then divide by 10.

In this scenario, you arrive at $119,500 for the average weighted EBIDTA. This is the number that is used as the benchmark by most corporate brokerage firms. They all take this number and apply a multiple to it. In the dental industry, it is common to have multiples of anywhere from 3 to 5.5. A multiple of 3 would indicate a practice that needs some updating in either equipment, technology, or both. This indicates the practice will need some investment from the buyer right at the time of the sale. As you move towards 4, this indicates the practice is already producing and collecting at a good rate. A practice with a valuation of 4 would need no major investment from the buyer. Typically a '4' practice is a very good practice that someone would be salivating to purchase. There have been sales of EBITDA multiples in the 4.5 to 6.5 range, but those are typically paid for by investors or corporate groups who have a plethora of free cash that needs to be invested. They tend to have private equity backing their financials, and are willing to pay more to enter a market they think is good. Above 4 is not a typical dental practice multiple in the single doctor practice category. See Table 1.3 for potential values for our example practice.

Table 1.3			
Multiple	3	3.5	4
Price	$358,500	$418,250	$478,000

After plugging the numbers into this table, we see that the value of this dental practice is anywhere between $358,000 and $478,000. This is quite a range! This is the starting point for the valuation. After assigning this valuation multiple, you assess things that are not in the calculation. Use the factors in the next section to determine whether the multiple should be closer to 3 or 4, or some other factor if there are other variables in play.

Other Factors in Practice Valuation

Here are some other factors in determining the value of a practice. Go through these questions to determine the answer for each point.

- Location:
    - Is the practice in a prime location?
    - What's the strength of the competition in the surrounding areas?
    - What are daily traffic numbers on the street outside the front door?
    - What is the number of rooftops in the 1-mile, 3-mile, and 5-mile radius?
    - What is the growth plan for the city around this location? Growing or stagnant?
- PPO participation:
    - How many PPO plans does the office take?
    - What percentage of patients are covered by which PPO plans?
    - What percentage of write-off do the PPO plans take off the usual and customary fees?
- Physical location:
    - Are you buying the building/space?
    - Are the lease or sale terms favorable for the buyer?
    - Number of operatories- Is there room for growth?
    - Age of building- Will there be higher repair costs in the future?
- Equipment:
    - Age and quality of equipment?
        - See chapter for inventory checklist
    - Will any equipment need to be updated?

- - Will there be any technology that needs updating?
- Staff Retention:
  - How many staff will be staying on?
  - What is the current compensation for the staff- above or below market rate?
- Procedures performed:
  - Does the doctor perform many procedures that are specialized in nature? Implants, full mouth reconstruction, molar root canals
  - Does the doctor do all their own hygiene?
  - Does the doctor already do a high volume of crowns? (Will all teeth be crowned prior to your arrival?)
- Patients
  - What is the number of active patients? (Seen in the last 18 months)
  - How many patients have had 2-3 prophy/perio maintenance in the last 18 months?
  - How many new patients per month?
  - Has the practice been net positive or negative on active patients? (Growing or shrinking practice?)
- Legal Issues
  - Is the seller set up as a PC, LLC, or C-Corp?
  - Are there any existing liens against the business?
  - Any liens against the building?
  - Any pending malpractice lawsuits?
  - Any other legal liabilities?

Once you as the buyer have your idea of perceived value, it is best to sit physically in the same room with the seller and discuss factors of valuation. It is not a good idea to approach this discussion from a viewpoint of disparaging the seller's practice, but to come to a mutual agreement on a price that works for both parties. Depending on whether the market is favorable for either the seller or the buyer, this can be a short discussion or a long one. You could be in agreement in an hour, or the negotiation could last for months. Remember, once the price is agreed upon, this is only the first step.

> To download and use a spreadsheet template to determine EBITDA value, go to addisonkilleen.com.
>
> Visit the website to find a list of vendors that may help with location search, demographics, PPO evaluation, practice statistics, and legal issues.

Allocation of Assets

The next step in the sale is the negotiation of what part of the price is allocated to fixed assets, 'blue sky', and the non-compete clause. This is important to discuss because it has different tax implications for the buyer and seller. Fixed assets are often called FF&E; for furniture, fixtures, and equipment. These are the things that could be carried out the door to a new location if you left a space. They can often be depreciated very quickly for tax purposes under current tax law.

The current law as of 2018 allows for a fixed asset to be depreciated instantly, for a value of up to $1,000,000 a year per entity. The buyer and seller should come to an agreement on which percentage allocation is given to equipment, which can usually be between 10-40% of the practice price. In certain situations where the practice is distressed, or has been unoccupied for a period of months, this percentage can approach 90%. FF&E also includes all the dental supplies and office supplies as well. If there are many computers or digital sensors, this would increase the percentage allocated to this.

It is advantageous for the seller to keep this amount as low as possible since the previous owner most likely already depreciated this asset down in value. They will have to pay a higher tax rate on this amount. For the buyer, it is desirable to set this as high as reasonably possible.

> Note: At the time of sale there should be two addenda to the contract. Addendum A should include all FF&E that is *included* in the sale. This list of included assets should be relatively exhaustive, but it doesn't need to go down the serial numbers on each chair or handpiece. Addendum B should list anything that is *not included* in the sale. Usually selling doctors want to take artwork or some items that have special value for them. Details in items like this can avoid having problems at the time of sale or immediately thereafter.

'Blue Sky', or goodwill, is the value of the patients walking in the door on a daily basis. This is often the largest allocation of the purchase price, as this is really where much of the value comes into play. For a seller, it is always better to have most of the value allocated to blue sky, as this is taxed at a lower rate for the seller. The buyer then has to amortize this cost over many years, which is not advantageous for the buyer. Arriving at this figure is a negotiation and there is no mathematical way to prove the value of 'Blue Sky'.

The last portion of the allocation price is a value to assign to a non-compete clause. Usually this is $5,000 to $15,000. If you are worried about a selling doctor going back into practice, it is very good to have a lawyer write a good non-compete clause. This clause can be very lenient or tough. The toughest, and quite common one, is that a value of $4,000 is given to each patient of record. Patient of record is usually defined as someone seen in the last 18 to 24 months. If the selling doctor was to move down the street and see that patient, then the selling doctor would have to pay the buyer $4,000 each time a former patient was seen. The value of the clause is tax favorable for the buyer, not the seller.

Below are a few examples of the allocations in recent sales:

Ex. 1	Total Price	$675,000	Annual Revenue $900k
	FF&E- $170,000	Goodwill- $500,000	Non-Compete- $5,000
Ex. 2	Total Price	$175,000	Annual Revenue $320k
	FF&E- $25,000	Goodwill- $150,000	Non-Compete- $0 (Doctor continued working)
Ex. 3	Total Price	$190,000	Annual Revenue $360k
	FF&E- $70,000	Goodwill- $110,000	Non-Compete- $10,000

Once you have negotiated all the allocations, this should be explicitly stated in the contract in a table. This is very important because when closing occurs, both parties will have to sign the IRS Form 8594 to let the IRS know that everyone was in agreement. That way after the sale, the IRS knows which parties in the transaction can claim the tax implications of blue sky and FF&E benefits.

To review, so far you should have these things done:

Valuation Checklist:
- 3 Years Tax Returns
- Input Data into EBITDA Spreadsheet
- Other Factors in Practice Valuation
    - Addendum of Included Equipment
    - Addendum of Excluded Equipment
- Determine EBITDA Multiple
- Allocation of Assets

After having these issues addressed, now it is time to look at some of the other decisions you will need to make when purchasing a practice.

Accounts Receivable

A common question when a selling doctor leaves a practice is whether they should hold onto any monies owed to them. Accounts Receivable (AR) are the totality of debts owed to the previous business by patients and insurers who are in the process of paying. There are three options for the AR:
- Purchase the AR
- Seller retains AR and buyer services it
- Seller retains AR and either services it themselves, or hires a 3rd party to do so

Purchase the AR

If the buyer purchases the AR, there should be a 'discount' applied to the amount due. Obviously many patients who felt obligated to pay their retiring doctor, may not feel the same way towards the new owner. This change in ownership may give that patient the needed nudge to stop paying. The other reason to pay a reduced fee on the AR is that it is going to cost the new owner time, postage, and energy to go after these people who, for one reason or another, were slow to pay the exiting doctor.

If you do purchase the AR, look closely at as many of the accounts as possible to know which discount percentages to assign to them. In general, here is a rule:

- 0-30 Days: Pay 85%
- 31-60 Days: Pay 80%
- 61-90 Days: Pay 50%
- Over 90 Days: Pay 30%

This is an average allocation of percentages and can be modulated depending on the circumstances and the goodwill that you think patients owe the selling doctor. When servicing this debt, it should appear that all debts are still being paid to the selling doctor. Letters should continue to come from the former dental practice, and patients should feel like they are still paying that doctor.

You can modulate the percentages based off historical trends, if they are available from the selling doctor. If the doctor has a very tight collections policy, maybe these percentages rise up towards 90% or 93% on the 0-30 Day AR. If the seller has a poor collections policy, with it taking more than 45 days to collect any money, then it might be better to move towards 80% or less.

The only advantage to this option is that all the collections that come in the door from day one go into the buyer's pocket. While there is an upfront cost to purchasing the AR, the ease of having cash-flow from the beginning is a good place to start. When financing, the bank will usually help with the entire cost, so the entire loan amount will include this AR. So even though you are paying interest on this, it can sometimes ease the headaches that come with slow cash-flow and transitions.

Selling doctors may feel slighted if they feel this is a 'low-ball' number. So you might consider the next option.

Seller Retains AR and Buyer Services It

In this option, the selling doctor maintains control and ownership of the AR. The Buyer then services it under the control of the purchased dental practice. In this case, it still appears that all debts are being paid to the dental practice and the selling doctor. The only difference is that after the money comes in, then the purchaser turns around and hands that money to the seller.

If going this route, it is important to include in the selling document a few 'rules of engagement'.
1. Limits on Actions: The buyer and seller should maintain and limit how aggressive they want to be in pursuing these accounts. There should be agreement that if an account is sent to a collection agency, that both parties are aware and informed of this fact.
2. First-In Money: If a patient owes money to a selling doctor and then gets service done with the new doctor, where does the first-in money go? Buyer and seller should agree on this scenario, but it usually means that seller gets their hand on this money first.
3. Collections Fee: After a certain number of days, either 30 or 45, then a 10-20% fee is assessed on all collections for the selling doctor. This way, the money that is already in the pipeline, either from insurance or checks in the mail, go 100% to the selling doctor. Any money that comes in after that date required some work by the buyer. In that case, the buyer should get paid a reasonable percentage for the work to collect that money.
4. End Date: After a certain date it becomes a nuisance to continue to maintain the seller's accounts. The remaining amount is typically very small. The buyer and seller should agree on an endpoint to the collections, so that there isn't an infinite timeline. Usually 6 months is appropriate. At that point, any accounts could be purchased out for a large discount, maybe 10-15% of amount.

The only downside to collecting for a selling doctor is that there is a lot of energy tied up in collecting and splitting out payments if you have a busy practice. Sometimes this can eat up a lot of energy from a staff that is already stressed by the change in ownership. Setting the ground rules from the beginning can ease a lot of the stress, and make sure that there isn't ill will between the parties after the sale.

Seller retains AR and services it

In this case, the seller will retain the AR. Sometimes a retiring dentist will take their book of accounts home and do it themselves, but more often their accountant will take care of it for them. Usually many patients will still mail checks to the practice or come to the practice to pay. In this case, you can keep a separate box for all payments, and then send this to the seller, or their accountant, as warranted.

There are many other small, but important, details to address in the sale or purchase of a practice. It is always a good idea to engage a knowledgeable legal team to help you address these issues.

> For more example documents, visit addisonkilleen.com to download them.

Financing

The banking and finance industry has historically seen dentists as good loan risks, and recent times haven't changed that much. Although it is getting harder to practice dentistry in a standalone office, banks will have no hesitation to lend to people who have their plan in place and are detailed in their analysis of the business. This next section will help you in gaining favorable financing whether you are buying an existing office or opening a new practice.

Buying a Practice

With any practice sale, the buyer is expecting that the historical revenues from the business will continue. Any financial institution being asked to finance the purchase will also want to see that this is the case. The good news is that in most cases where there is a smooth transition of business, almost 90% of all patients get retained. Most of the time, banks know about business transition, but it is best to approach them with a lot of information so that you show you are an expert before asking for financing.

When you approach a bank, you will want to figure out the entire cost you will need to purchase this practice, or start up this practice. This includes, but may not be limited to:
- Purchase Price of practice
- Purchase of Accounts Receivable (Money owed to selling dentist)
- Money (Capital) needed for new equipment/upgrades
- Working Capital (Money needed to run business until you generate profit)

For an example, let's examine the purchase of a practice for $175,000. In this example, you might also be purchasing the Accounts Receivable for $31,000. The entire AR was potentially $40,000. Once the discount is applied to the entire amount, the sale price for the AR will be $31,000. Since the seller was woefully out of date with technology and equipment, let's say you have set up a schedule to spend $90,000 on digital records, digital radiology, a pantomograph, marketing, and new dental supplies. Since you purchased the AR, you may not need any line of credit. The total for this loan package would then be $296,000. (See the following table.)

Sales Price	$175,000
Accounts Receivable	$31,000
Working Capital	$0
Equipment, Technology, Updating	$90,000
TOTAL	$296,000

What will you need to prepare for the initial financing request? When you approach a bank, you should be very detailed about everything you do. Here is the list of items it will be important to have ready in a packet for any financial institution you will approach for financing:
1. Sale price, Accounts Receivable (if purchasing), and any investments needed to be made immediately
2. Working capital (if needed)- sometimes called Line of Credit
3. Pro Forma Statement
4. Personal Financial Statement of each member in purchasing practice

After showing the bank all expected expenses, the bank will want to know what percentage of the entire sales price needs financing. If the buyer needs 100% financing, sometimes terms become less favorable. The interest rate usually rises quite significantly when you approach 100% total financing.

More institutions will give you favorable terms for financing at the 80% level. Now this doesn't mean 80% of just the purchase price, but the entire loan package. At $296,000 for the total purchase price in the example, 80% financing would be a loan for $236,800. This means that a buyer would have to bring $59,200 to the sale.

Working Capital

If this practice is a startup or you are not purchasing the Accounts Receivable, it is almost always necessary to have a cash account to draw upon to pay the bills until the business produces enough money to cash flow. This access to money is called working capital or a line of credit.

It is sometimes a guessing game as to how much working capital will be needed during a transition, but it is always better to guess high and not need as much. The bank may not respond favorably if you have to come back and ask for a higher limit.

In principle, working capital is money that you will borrow from the bank to pay for operating expenses. You will repay only interest during the duration that the money is borrowed. If the working capital account is only accessed for $10,000 for a duration of 30 days, then the business will be charged the daily interest rate on that money for the month it is borrowed. If the practice needs up to $50,000 over the course of a year, then that is a lot more interest paid. Arriving at how much working capital is needed is a complicated guess, but a pro forma will be useful in determining a safe amount.

Pro Forma Statement

> Definition: The *pro forma* models the anticipated results of the transaction, with particular emphasis on the projected cash flows, net revenues and taxes. Consequently, *pro forma* statements summarize the projected future status of a company, based on the current financial statements.

A pro forma statement looks a lot like what the books might look like after the first year in business, with each month in a column across the top, and all cost categories down the left side. The pro forma statement is a forward-looking anticipation of income, cost, and net profit before taxes, depreciation, and amortization.

Creating a pro forma statement is not too difficult from a high level view. Be aware that there will be many assumptions, and not all assumptions will be correct, or even close in some circumstances.

It is best, if buying a current practice, to use the historical numbers to anticipate future numbers. As long as the wages/salaries of employees aren't going to be changed, then keep those numbers the same for the first year. If the buyer knows of cost savings or areas to improve the business, add those in and decrease the expenses. The bank financing the transaction will be happy to know that the buyer will make the business more profitable than historical numbers.

> Go to addisonkilleen.com- Resources to find a good example of a pro forma and a clean document you can use when creating a new pro forma statement.

Anticipating income and costs during a transition is one of the trickiest parts of a pro forma. For a dental startup, it is important to anticipate that income will be slow to come in. You are building a patient base from scratch, and there is not an existing Accounts Receivable in the pipeline. Another reason is that any PPO plan you join will be slow in credentialing. This can sometimes take up to 90 days before you become 'in-network'. Only once you get that designation will your claims be processed. Usually all PPOs back-date their approval of the dentist so that a patient seen on opening day of a practice gets the PPO rate, but you will want to confirm this directly with each carrier.

Typically there is a little bit of a lag in collections, and sometimes this is due to the collections policy the buyer has versus the outgoing seller. Many long-standing doctors may have had lenient collections policies, which allowed patients to just, "Pay when you get the bill from us." This is a poor way of doing business for many reasons, but it also makes it harder on the buyer. When the new buyer comes in, makes the investment in all new technology and brings the practice up to date, they will often have a more strict policy on collections which will be: Pay the patient portion the day of service. This can sometimes create friction with longstanding patients of the practice, but it is a short-lived pain for long-term gain. Creating a comprehensive plan for financing, and making sure all patients are aware of their financial responsibilities, will create a more open environment and lead to better financial health for the buyer and the business.

During the first 6 months of a transition, anticipate that the Accounts Receivable will most likely go up and month to month production/collections will be somewhat variable. This increase in the AR will be due to insurance issues and getting patients acclimated to the new owner's collections philosophy. Production and collections month to month will also be variable due to having to build up a rapport with patients and having some patients wait on treatment that they would otherwise have completed. Due to these two issues, it is best to make all revenue forecasts very conservative, and anticipate a good amount of working capital so that you can feel financially secure during the transition.

As for all costs on the pro forma, plan on keeping all costs in line with what the selling doctor was paying. To be safe, all costs could even be inflated and increased to show any bank that you are making the most conservative estimates available. If you are a disciple of the numbers, and I hope that you are, then you should anticipate over time that you will get **your lab bill down to 6% of revenues and your dental supplies to 4% of revenues.** This may not be possible during the transition months, mostly due to having to upgrade any supplies that you want and feel comfortable with. After about 3-4 months, however, this should be achievable.

The process of going through the pro forma also gives the buyer the opportunity to really understand all the costs of the practice. Take this opportunity to scrutinize every cost category and ask all the 'Why?' questions. Why do we pay for an automated call service? Why do we pay for a person to come in and clean the office? Asking all these questions will lead you to become a better business person, and in turn, lead banks to feel more comfortable about loaning money to you.

Personal Financial Statement

Many banks will have their own Personal Financial Statement (PFS) form that they would like the borrower to use. It is best that the buyer be one step ahead and have this completed prior to approaching the bank. The general outline is:
1. Assets
    a. Checking Accounts
    b. Savings Accounts
    c. Stock/Bond accounts not held in retirement/tax-advantaged accounts
    d. Retirement Accounts- usually not, but can be included for full disclosure
2. Liabilities
    a. Student Loans
    b. Other loans for any other items
3. Real Estate
    a. Value of any real estate
    b. Loans owed against that property
    c. Liens against the property
4. Vehicles
    a. Current value of any vehicles, boats, etc.
    b. Loans against those vehicles
5. Business Interests
    a. Current value of any shares
    b. Current loans against any shares

Once all this documentation is put together, it is best to print this off on high quality paper, put it into a 3-ring binder or nice packet, and then hand-deliver to each banking institution that you are approaching for financing. In the world of government, 3 bids are required for any project, and you should follow the same rule. Go to 3 separate banks and ask for their best terms.

Startup Documents and Plan

Many books have been written about doing a dental startup- and I would suggest if you're taking this route that you should read every one of them. There are too many little pieces to a startup to address in one chapter, and so we will just look at the Financing portion of them here. The bank will need the same 4 items:

1. Initial Capital
    a. Tenant Improvements to a rented space (Even if you own the building)
    b. FF&E- Furniture, Fixtures, and Equipment
    c. Dental supplies at startup
    d. Office supplies
    e. Marketing budget (from 5. Marketing Plan)
2. Working capital (if needed)- sometimes called Line of Credit
3. Pro Forma Statement
4. Personal Financial Statement
5. Marketing Plan

Initial Capital

The Initial capital is the bulk of the loan you may need to do a *de novo*, or startup dental office. This capital can be separated into a few major categories.

The Tenant improvements are changes that you make to a space that make it a dental office. This includes the plumbing, cabinets, and work areas that will make it usable. If you own the building, you will separate out the costs of purchasing, or constructing, the shell of the office, and all other costs. This makes a huge difference for the depreciation schedule that you can apply to different aspects of the building. The shell is the roofing, siding, concrete, and main structure of the building- all the way down to the studs. This has a long lifespan, and so the IRS wants to allow you to depreciate it over many years.

The tenant finish, however, can reasonably be said to have a shorter lifespan. Depending on the tax law during the year you build, you may be able to depreciate the entire tenant finish during one year. This cost can be paid by the business loan, and depreciated faster. Items included in the tenant finish would be carpet, drywall, some plumbing, some electrical, tile, bathroom fixtures, built-in desks, built-in cabinetry, doors, and any woodwork. All of these costs should be included in the initial capital for the tenant improvements. It is best to itemize all these costs in as much detail as possible for the loan request so that the bank knows you are an expert.

> Tip: Cities often have Tax Increment Finance (TIF) dollars, or other economic development programs, to help with redevelopment of what is considered 'blighted' or underserved areas. This doesn't always mean these areas are truly ugly or run-down, it only means that the city's economic development arm will support redevelopment with tax dollars on the front end of a project. It is best to check with the local city offices to see what programs are available.

FF&E

The next category you will need to identify is furniture, fixtures, and equipment. Office furniture and other small things can add up. You will need to choose wisely what is best for your startup budget. Sometimes office furniture can be quite expensive, and you should be ready to shop for bargains in that area. All other office supplies and computers should be budgeted and planned for in this category as well.

The biggest cost in FF&E is dental equipment. This is always what blows up your budget because of the high initial cost of ownership of dental equipment. Compressors, suction pumps, handpieces, dental units, and x-ray tubes are quite expensive. It is best to have an idea of what you want to pay, and then approach a few different vendors asking for bids. Equipment like this has a large markup, so they have room to come down to your budget if necessary.

> Tip from Michael Lomotan of Divergent Dental: "Call all of the big distributors and have them come in to provide you with a full equipment list. Go for the whole package, then start trading quotes to get to the lowest possible bid. Once that's done, you piece it out, remove what you don't need, and get individual bids from other vendors."

There are also vendors that have used equipment on the internet. This can sometimes be a safe place to purchase equipment, but then you will need a service technician or someone else to install and maintain them. Buying chairs, dental carts and lights would be advisable from one of these vendors, but compressors and suction pumps are a bad idea. For the equipment that has to be up 100% of the time for your office to be open, it is best not to buy used equipment.

> Note: Sometimes equipment manufacturers will give more favorable loan terms, like 0% interest for 5 years, because they already make their money on the equipment. This could reduce the amount of money you'd need from a bank.

Computers, sensors, and technology can also be a big part of your budget. This will be a huge and complicated decision, so you will need to do a lot of research before purchasing any of this. Another large decision will be whether you run your practice management software off a server or the cloud. A server can run anywhere up to $5,000. Also plan on having TVs or multiple computer screens in any operatory. It is usually best to have a good technology company that specializes in dental offices help you come to these decisions.

Dental Supplies

This cost category can sometimes be large during a startup phase, but it doesn't have to be. It is best to get a small baseline of supplies, and then only order when needed. Currently, you can order something from the big distributors and have all the supplies delivered within 48 hours. This means that you really don't need to have more than a couple of days' worth of supplies on hand at any one time. This reduction in dental supplies means you can have more money in your pocket, not sitting on your shelves.

Marketing Budget

In this economy, there is almost no way that you can just open your doors and have a successful business. There is too much competition and cut-throat marketing for you to just open a location on a busy corner and expect to be inundated with patients. At first, and probably forever, you will need a marketing plan. This means that you will need to invest a decent amount of money to have both a passive presence and an active presence in your market.

Passive presence would be your website, digital footprint, and signage. Engage a good dental-specific marketing firm to have a website where, if people look for you, they will find out about you. This will be the same with Facebook, Google+, and every other platform. No matter if you want to be aggressive about going out and pushing content, you will at least need to be there if a patient comes looking. This cost category also includes hard signage on your building or out by the street. This means that when patients actually come looking for you, they can find you. Sometimes these are large investments, but they will last many years and are a necessity.

Active presence on the marketing front is usually less fun. This means mailing postcards, buying billboards, doing Facebook Ads, Google Ads, and spending money in other ways to catch patients who otherwise don't know you exist, or know they need you. The return on investment for many of these things is sometimes small, but at the beginning they are necessary to get a critical mass of patients.

It is important to note that a decent marketing budget is not to be overlooked. The standard marketing expense is 5 percent of revenues. If your goal is to collect $700,000 in your first year, then you should plan on at least $35,000 in marketing during that year, and that is not including the baseline costs of a good website, signage, and other starting materials.

Startup Financial Checklist:
1. Initial Capital
    a. Tenant Improvements or Construction
    b. FF&E- Furniture, Fixtures, and Equipment
    c. Dental Supplies
    d. Office Supplies
    e. Marketing budget
2. Working Capital
3. Pro Forma Statement
4. Personal Financial Statement
5. Marketing Plan

The total of all the initial capital needed for a startup may surprise you. When seeing what the payments can be on a large loan like this, you may think there is a good chance of failure. The good news is that only .4% of dentists ever go into bankruptcy, so there's a really good chance that success is more likely than failure.

Once you have the initial capital portion detailed, then you continue with the next 3 items-- a figure for working capital, your Pro Forma Statement, and your Personal Financial Statement. Put this into a nice package and shop it around to 3 financial institutions. Just filling out all the paperwork will feel like success, but the fun part is actually getting the practice off the ground. Thoroughly doing all the detailed work at the beginning will only lead to further financial success down the road.

Legal Issues and Taxes

Whether you are buying or starting a dental practice, you deserve the very best professional advice. The importance of having good lawyers and accountants cannot be understated. Finding a team that specializes in dentistry can be difficult or time-consuming, but the special knowledge they bring can save many hundreds of thousands of dollars down the road.

What follows is just a high-level overview of some of the issues and ways to minimize your headaches as you start your journey. Check with a local attorney for regulations in your state, as many state laws dictate the best course strategy.

Limited Liability Corporation

Most dental offices should be established as a Limited Liability Corporation (LLC), filing taxes as an S Corporation. This means the practice is formed as a closely held corporation that passes through all income, or losses, to its shareholders. In these cases, the owners claim this income on their personal income tax forms

and they pay tax at the personal income rate. To be an S Corporation, you must:
- Have no more than 100 shareholders
- All Shareholders are individual persons,
- Have only one class of stock.

When forming an LLC, you will need a legal team to apply for a name, draft all documents, and assign stock membership to any owners. If it is just a one-person company, then that one owner owns 100% of the stock.

> Tip: Sometimes your legal counsel will also suggest a Professional Limited Liability Corporation, or a PLLC. This may offer some other legal protections, although seek the counsel of an attorney for the best option.

Your first LLC will own the dental business. This can be named the same as your dental practice, and it is basically your main company.

You may also want a second LLC for any real estate you own. You will want to form this LLC, and name it anything under the sun, and pay yourself market-rate rent from your dental business into this LLC. This provides a firewall against any unwanted legal troubles. If someone slips and hurts themselves on the sidewalk, they can sue the property LLC, but it will be harder to sue the dental business. Same thing going the other way: if someone sues your dental practice, they will have a harder time gaining access to any of your property income when the property is in a different LLC. Another advantage is that tax law is favorable towards property, which an accountant will advise on.

C Corporation

A C-Corporation is an entity where the income is taxed at the corporation level, and not passed through to the personal level. So after the business makes or loses money, it is taxed before being passed out as dividends.

This usually presents a poor value proposition for any dental practices, as you will pay taxes twice before getting to take any money home. The first tax is the corporate profit tax, and then if you pay out dividends to shareholders, it is taxed a second time at a different rate. It is for this reason that the C-Corp is almost never used and should be avoided in dentistry. However, check with your tax advisor as tax laws change frequently.

Tax Issues

The job of a good accountant is to make sure you pay the taxes for which you are liable, and not more. Finding the right corporate structure is the first key to making sure you are paying appropriate taxes, but there are many other steps you need to get right.

Maximize Depreciation

Depreciation is the *"reduction in the value of an asset with the passage of time, due in particular to wear and tear."* This can either be in reference to the tax side of depreciation or the actual operational wear and tear on any asset. After you purchase an asset, you can usually use a depreciation table to figure out how much value the asset lost in any given year. Remember that this depreciation amount becomes a cost that reduces net income, and thereby reduces tax liability. It is not real money, only a line item that helps with taxes.

Let's assume you buy a piece of equipment, a Cone Beam-CT machine, for $100,000. A high-tech piece of equipment like this is usually almost obsolete in 3 to 5 years. Due to this fact, the IRS will usually allow you to say that the asset lost value over the course of either 3 or 5 years. Your accountant will be able to help classify this cost, but in general, you want to depreciate it as fast as possible. Table A-1 shows the percentages of depreciation that an asset can experience during each year of its lifespan.

Table A-1

Year	Depreciation Rate- Property Half-year Convention					
	3-Year	5-Year	7-Year	10-Year	15-Year	20-year
1	33.33%	20.00%	14.29%	10.00%	5.00%	3.750%
2	44.45	32.00	24.4	18.00	9.50	7.219
3	14.81	19.20	17.49	14.40	8.55	6.667
4	7.41	11.52	12.49	11.52	7.70	6.177
5		11.52	8.93	9.22	6.93	5.713
6		5.76	8.92	7.37	6.23	5.285
7			8.93	6.55	5.90	4.88
8			4.46	6.55	5.90	4.522
9				6.56	5.91	4.462
10				6.55	5.90	4.461
11				3.28	5.91	4.462
12					5.90	4.461
13					5.91	4.462
14					5.90	4.461
15					5.91	4.462
16					2.95	4.461
17						4.462
18						4.461
19						4.462
20						4.461
21						2.231

Internal Revenue Service, 2017

In recent years, Congress has almost always instituted Section 179. Sec. 179 of the tax code allows for any purchase up to $250,000 to be depreciated all in one year. Typically, if you buy a piece of equipment with the profits from a given year, then you have to pay your normal tax rate on those profits first. So, let's say you made $100,000 in profits in a given year. After taxes take 38%, then you have only $62,000 to potentially buy any assets.

However, if Sec. 179 is in place during that tax year, then you will be able to claim any depreciation, totaling up to $250,000, all in one year. So if you purchased a CBCT, and you depreciate the entire amount in a single year, you avoid paying the $38,000 in taxes on that $100,000. It is as if the US Federal Government will purchase for you about 40% of any new equipment up to $250,000 during a single year.

You might be thinking, this is absolutely crazy for the Federal Government to do this. Depends on your stance, but in general the US Congress has believed that this Sec. 179 in the tax code has encouraged lots of investment by small businesses, and that is worth the cost in lost tax revenue.

So, in general, if you spend less than $250,000 on equipment during a single year, then you will be able to take the entire cost of the equipment as a tax 'loss'. If you spend more than $250,000, then you will have to refer to the original percentage on the depreciation schedule in Table A-1.

Real Estate Depreciation

Many times dentists will own their real estate as well as their practice. Most tax planning professionals will say that a piece of commercial real estate will depreciate over 39.5 years. To calculate this depreciation, make sure you separate the value of the building from the value of the land. The IRS legally says that the land is not depreciable, but that the building will depreciate fully over 39.5 years. That means that every year, you will take 2.53% depreciation over the course of 39.5 years.

Let's say that a property was purchased for $250,000. The land is worth $100,000 and the building is worth $150,000. For every year for the life of the building, you can take a 2.53% loss on the building portion, or $3,795 per year.

The way to accelerate depreciation is ask your accountant for a segregation study. In a segregation study, your accountant or tax advisor will take your building and divide its value into sub-categories like:

- Site Work
- Concrete & Masonry: Sidewalks, foundation, flooring
- Steel: Shell of the building
- Woods & Plastics: Finish woodwork, cabinetry, rough carpentry
- Thermal & Moisture Protection: Roofing, insulation,
- Doors & Windows
- Specialties: Dental cabinetry, dental lighting, restrooms, lockers
- Finish: Carpet, paint
- Mechanical
- Electrical

After you have a segregation study completed, you can then look to depreciate some of these areas faster than the 39.5 years. Items like the Electrical can potentially be depreciated in 15 years. Carpet and paint will wear out in 5 to 7 years. In this scenario, you can accelerate the depreciation schedule to get more depreciation in the early years of property ownership. This means more money in your pocket in the early years of property ownership.

Tax Strategy

A smart business owner will try to take legal advantage of anything they can to make sure they pay the least amount in taxes, and thereby re-invest any possible capital into the business. Some accountants will be able to help with many of these things, but it is incredibly important to find a good accountant who has a good knowledge about the dental industry to be able to help in all facets of the business. Here are a few of the items to review with your tax professional:

- Management Company: There are some benefits to having an 'upstream' management company. This is a wholly-owned LLC above all other subsidiary LLCs. There are potential write-offs and avenues to decrease tax liability inside a management company that are not possible inside your dental practice. Ask your tax planning professional if there are any ways to use a management company that may help you decrease your liability.

- Vehicle allowance: Your business can rightfully pay for a portion of your vehicle if you use your personal vehicle to do some tasks for the business. Discuss with your accountant the best way to pay for a portion of the vehicle through the company.

- Meals and Entertainment: It is possible that you, as a business owner, may occasionally buy food for your staff or patients if you see them at the local watering hole. This is also the same if you are meeting a dental classmate and sharing tips on how to run your practices better.

- Cell Phone and Internet: In this day and age, having a cell phone is a necessity for a dentist. We are on call for our patients much of the time. It is right and just that we run our cell phone bill through the practice. If we have a 'Home Office', it is also right that we can pay for a portion of our home internet, to work on payroll, accounting, statistics, and completing patients' charts at night.

- Home Office: You probably use your home for a 'home office' for some time of the working week. As long as it's 10-12 hours per week, the IRS will allow the expense of an office at your residence. One way is to add up all the square feet of the office, and then find a market rate per sq. ft. per year. The other way is called the 'Safe Harbor' method. The IRS has made a normalized way to pay rent to your residence, and this is $5 for up to 300 Sq. Ft. of your home. So the total in this scenario is to pay $1,500 to yourself each year for rent.

- Renting your Home: Did you know it is legal for you to rent your own house for work events up to 14 days a year at a normal market rate? Ask for 3 competing bids from local establishments on a room rental, and then you are legally allowed to rent your house, from yourself, for up to 14 days per year for work events. When you get competing bids, try to shoot for times of the year or dates that may be at the higher end of the spectrum. Check with your CPA before counting this as a business expense, as it is becoming increasingly scrutinized.

- Travel: Many times there are CE courses offered in distant and exotic locations. These trips can be written off if they are considered "ordinary and necessary" to run your dental business. If you choose to take your spouse, their flight may not be a necessary business expense, but the hotel room for you is surely ordinary and necessary.

- <u>Other business expenses:</u> Remember that any item or asset that is used for business, can legally be purchased by the business.

In general, taxes are a part of life. You will have to pay them, and most likely you will have to pay quite a substantial amount. The key to being successful is using the tax code to your advantage to pay the correct amount, and not to overpay. This is why it is incredibly important to shop around for advisors and an accountant who can help you minimize your taxes, by the rules, as smart as possible. There's nothing more painful at the end of the day than knowing that you paid more tax than was necessary.

Watching the Numbers

> *Most people use statistics the way a drunkard uses a lamp post, more for support than illumination."*
> – Mark Twain

I've met a few dentists in recent years who are just frustrated. For many dentists incomes have been flat since the 2008 Stock Market slump. With the inflation rate, however small, this actually means the buying power of your income has actually decreased. In the field of dentistry, there is no shortage of reasons to be concerned.

A while back, I met with a dentist who was looking at his numbers. He was about to buy out a retiring doctor, and he had never actually seen the Profit and Loss statement until it came time to complete the purchase of the practice. As it turns out, the practice owner was actually losing $80,000 a year to keep the practice afloat and to employ the associate! As the transition was to occur very soon, this was an absolute disaster. Many options were on the table, including walking away from a great patient base. This was a demoralizing situation.

We met a few times and talked through the ways to hit targets, and implement systems. After working through the benchmark numbers that the practice needed to hit, this dentist took control of the day to day management of the practice. The patients were great, but the previous owner was just spending money and not keeping track of where it went.

After this trial period of management by the statistics, the practice showed a profit of a few thousand the first month. Then $5,000 the second month. By the end of the third month, the profits were nearly $10,000 for the month. Once this new dentist took control of the numbers, he was on track to have the practice show a profit of almost $100,000 that year. This was above paying himself a wage to do the dentistry!

Before going into how we can fix problems like this, I want to tell a story of the Hawthorne Works plant outside Cicero, Illinois. In 1924, there was a study commissioned by the Hawthorne executives:

> The Hawthorne Works had commissioned a study to see if their workers would become more productive in higher or lower levels of light.

As the researchers were watching the productivity, they started to change the variable in the equation- the lighting level. At first they raised the lighting level. This led to an overall increase in productivity. The researchers were delighted, and thought that they had found the solution! Just to be sure however, they started to lower the lighting level to see if it would cause a decrease in productivity. To their surprise, it increased the productivity even more!

This Hawthorne Effect, as it is called, reveals an important fact that when people are being monitored or measured, they feel empowered to modify their behavior. This is the same thing that you can leverage in your dental practice. Once you start watching the statistics, you will be able to get your employees to become more productive, you can help your staff to be more engaged with patients, and you can see your overall business become a well-oiled machine.

So now you understand the need to gather statistics on every facet of your practice, but you don't know what to do next. That is okay. The first step is to gather the baseline data and look at benchmarks from other practices. After doing that, you will be able to make informed decisions that will increase the productivity and profitability of your practice.

To illustrate this, look at what recently happened in one of my practices. I had set a new goal for the practice to reduce the No Show/Late Cancel rate (NS/CX). I had my staff look at this statistic every day, measure it, and put it on a cloud-based spreadsheet. After doing this for a few weeks, the staff started seeing how high our rate was- almost 9.5% of appointments were being missed or cancelled on the day of appointment. This left us with open chair time and decreased production.

After watching this for 3 weeks, my staff was disheartened. They felt disrespected by patients who wouldn't come to their appointments. They came up with a solution without any input from me. The idea is described later in this book. We implemented their suggestion over the course of 2 months, and we have consistently dropped our No Show/Cancel (NS/CX) percentage by nearly 2%. I won't claim that my office runs as well as it could, but any gain is a huge increase in production and profits, not to mention the satisfaction of the staff. Changing this NS/CX rate by 2% over the course of an $800k practice could mean as much as $16,000 more dollars in your pocket. Will you watch the data for $16,000? What if watching the data could make a $100,000 swing in your yearly income?

Why is this story important? It shows that sometimes you don't even need to motivate your staff to do anything different. Once you have the data, and some benchmarks, your staff will want to hit those marks to know that they are playing with a successful team. No one likes to be on a mediocre or losing team.

In the dental field, we want everyone in the population to be able to have a dental home, and we know that we capture only 50% of the market! So by having your office win, that doesn't mean the office down the street is necessarily losing anything. We just want every office to be functioning at a high level, playing at the 'Pro' level. By watching the numbers, engaging your staff in the data, you will see changes and ideas will come that you never thought possible.

Leading Indicators and Key Production Indicators

Leading Indicators (LIs) will be able to tell you a week or month in advance where you can expect your production to be headed. Key Production Indicators are the trailing indicators of the work you've already completed. This is a major theme of the book, *The 4 Disciplines of Execution* by Chris McChesney, Sean Covey, and Jim Huling. They look at leading indicators that can focus your energy on achieving the biggest KPI, a *wildly important goal* (WIG). The leading indicators listed here are the most useful and impactful when trying to run your dental practice better.

KPIs, or Key Production Indicators, are more of a lag indicator, telling the story of what has already happened. KPIs are often the hot words in dentistry and business, and these are important to know because you can set your major goals on the KPIs. LIs, on the other hand, are what will help you achieve your goals.

When looking at indicators or statistics of your practice, it is important that any number should be able to lead you toward a decision about the operation of your practice. You should have control over the items being measured. It's great to measure everything, but if you're measuring something over which you have no control, then it's a waste of your time. You could measure everything in your practice down to how much water you use every month, but it's an exercise in futility if you don't have any control over the outcome.

Another problem that we have is that the availability of the numbers determines what we see. We then tend to overestimate the importance of the information we have at hand, while missing the big picture. If production is an easy number to always see, we start to put more weight in that number than any other.

Recent psychological articles also point to the fact that too much data induces paralysis. If you start watching too many points, then you will get lost in what we call, "analysis paralysis". If you think that you can correlate 500 data points to point you in a singular direction, then you will be searching for eternity. However, if you use the 15 most important points, then usually they will lead you in the direction that make the most business sense. A 'Scorecard' as the Harvard Business School teaches, should be simple enough that you could read it on a beach somewhere in a couple minutes, and get a total picture of the health of your business.

Unfortunately, in the business of dentistry, we have to be the ones in the office producing to make any money, but you get the idea. So after we get that beach idea out of our heads, let's move on to the most important statistics that you need to watch in your practice.

Why Leading Indicators?

Leading indicators are the most important thing to watch because they tell you how your business is going to do before you can read it in the daily production numbers. As comedian Steve Harvey says, "You can't drive a car looking in the rear view mirror!" While he says this to be funny, this is what many dentists do on a day to day basis. While they don't address every system in the practice, these leading indicators will give you the best overall picture of how the numbers will go in the future.

These indicators are split into categories to watch weekly and monthly. Weekly numbers are things you can change very quickly with feedback, while monthly numbers are slower to change and can be calculated once a month.

Weekly LIs

Number of Days to Next New Patient Appointment

In your practice, you will have a set appointment length for a new patient exam and prophy. Sometimes this can be 60 minutes, but most often it is 90 minutes or more. In our group we often call this the 'Rock' in the hygiene schedule. A Rock is a 90-minute block that can either hold a new patient or 2 quadrants of Scaling and Root planing. Either way, the 'Rock' appointment time usually leads to some high production relative to a regular prophy appointment. It also usually leads to filling the Doctor's schedule with important work.

In addition, this number is important because it lets you know when you have reached capacity for your hygiene department. If you are adding many new patients a month, sometimes this can cause a new patient to be scheduled for his or her return visit too far into the future. If a patient isn't really set on coming to you, but rather just looking for anyone near their house, then they might go elsewhere if you are booking 2-3 weeks away.

The goal for the number of days to the next available new patient appointment should be less than 7 days. If someone figures out, "Hey I need to get into a dentist for a cleaning and exam," dentistry is at the top of their mind for that moment. If you are going to schedule them more than 7 days out, then they have a higher chance of not showing up, or finding another dentist who can schedule them more quickly. If you start having an average of more than 7 days for a new patient, consider adding hygiene time to increase capacity.

There is another advantage to having this number below 7 days. Usually this 90 minute block will be used by a new patient, but if you are treatment planning within normal limits, it can also be used by Scaling and Root planing patients as well. If you are booking too far in advance for these ScRP patients, they will not accept the urgency of the situation, and may have a higher rate of not showing up for the appointment.

Number of Days to Next Doctor Rock Appointment

Just like a hygiene rock appointment described before, this is the number of days until a large opening in the doctor's schedule. A Rock appointment for the doctor would be usually around 90 minutes where the doctor can do a lengthy or complex procedure. This could be a crown and some fillings, or just an entire quadrant of fillings. Such high dollar production would usually take care of a significant amount of the daily doctor goal production, potentially $1,500 or more.

If this number starts to average above the comfort zone of 7 days, then look for ways to add capacity or times earlier than 7 days. This could mean adding an assistant to open up another available room per day, or you may want to evaluate whether your patient flow warrants adding another associate dentist in the practice, if space allows.

If the doctor is already running 2 chairs simultaneously and a few hygienists every day, then there may not be time to add another doctor. If adding another assistant is possible to help run another operatory, this is usually the best return-on-investment. This could be an assisted hygiene routine, or a 3rd room for the Doctor's patients. Adding an associate is much more complicated and can only be done with a high new patient flow, or some other major change in the office.

Fluoride Rate

The benefits of fluoride have been recognized over the years. This has been proven by many researchers, and the American Dental Association has reiterated many times the importance of water fluoridation and topical fluoride. Newer research has continued to support the use of fluoride, and now supports the use of topical fluoride in adults. For those in the 'Moderate to High Risk' category for caries, the ADA recommends that we place a fluoride varnish every 6 months.

We all know those patients who are at a moderate to high risk. Sometimes you can see it from 5 feet away! Basically, we need to make sure we give every patient the chance to keep their natural teeth in the most conservative way. We try to get this fluoride percentage over 90% every day.

Some insurances cover fluoride for the life of the patient, but many do not. If you have control over pricing, keep the prices at a moderate rate to encourage close to 100% usage for those who need it. Remember that a fluoride varnish usually costs between $1-$2.25 per application, so setting the price at a market rate of $10-30 is a win almost every time.

Sometimes your practice management software will track your fluoride rate. If you don't use a software that can, you can use a simple grid on paper to track it. The example on the right can be printed onto a ¼ size sheet of paper. This can then be kept by each hygienist every day to keep track of the statistic.

Monday	Hygienist:	
	Received Fluoride	Re-Appoint?
1		
2		
3		
4		
5		
6		
7		
8		
9		
Total		

CX/NS Rate

This is the rate of patients who are on the schedule, but either cancel their appointment within 24 hours or just don't show up. This rate can really kill the production in the office, and it hurts worst in hygiene because you miss the opportunity to plan for treatment for any other services.

Some offices routinely have about 9%-12% of patients either cancel late or fail to show up. This means you are still paying to have the lights on and staff ready, but have zero income. Some consultants will say you can get this number down to 3% or less. I would say that if you are even down to 4%, then you will be doing a great job.

As I mentioned in the introduction, tracking this number will lead to potential ideas for changes in behavior. There are consulting organizations that teach very effective strategies to reduce this percentage. Using an automated service to text or call your patients can also be great. Look for all the different products out there that may work with your practice management system to see what may work best.

Your staff can also help by coming up with good ideas to reduce this number. One of the things my staff came up with recently is to email patients the morning of their appointment. We had already been tracking this percentage for a while, and we thought that some people just plain forgot they had an appointment. We all understand; kids' sports activities, projects due at work, and any other number of things. So we tried an email the morning of, about 7:30am, saying:

> Hello John,
> We really look forward to seeing you for your appointment today at 1pm!
>
> Thanks,
> Your Dental Team

To say this was a success is an understatement. Through this simple and free method, we reduced the CX/NS rate by a significant amount! The great thing was that the staff came up with the idea, and implemented it. After trying it for a few weeks we could see the average dropping and the staff was elated. They now have a feeling of ownership from helping to improve the rate.

Forward Production Target

This forward gross production target is always looking 7 days in the future. First, the office manager should take the planned production for the next 7 days, and put that into the spreadsheet. You will already have the production goal for the next 7 days, or ¼ of the month. That production goal will normally be stable, but you could modulate it if you know you're taking a vacation or will be down a staff member. Then, you look at what percent of the goal is currently planned, or scheduled. This could be 60%, this could be 105%. At 60%, this means you will need to do some same-day dentistry to catch up. At 105%, this could mean that your office manager is hitting the goal and scheduling very well to hit the goal.

Each week you will chart this on a spreadsheet like the one below. If the numbers look good, as in a high percentage over 85%, then color the space green. If the numbers look to be in the mid-range, then color the square yellow. If the numbers are looking low, or below 65%, then color the square red. Obviously we don't like seeing red, and we like seeing green.

> Hint: Use the conditional formatting feature in Excel, where the numbers will actually color themselves after you enter the data. You will enter the parameters, and Excel will change the fill color of the cell automatically.

Date	End Date		Ending Production
4/24/2017	5/1/2017	**$17,871**	
	Goal	$15,976	
	% of Goal	**111.86%**	$18,348
	Fill Avg.	78.96%	114.85%
5/1/2017	5/8/2017	**$10,526**	
	Goal	$15,976	
	% of Goal	**65.89%**	$12,849
	Fill Avg.	78.96%	80.43%
5/8/2017	5/15/2017	**$8,340**	
	Goal	$15,976	
	% of Goal	**52.20%**	$14,256
	Fill Avg.	78.96%	89.23%
5/15/2017	5/22/2017	**$15,618**	
	Goal	$15,976	
	% of Goal	97.76%	$16,385
	Fill Avg.	**78.96%**	102.56%

When we plot these forward looking numbers in the 3rd column, we also plot the previous week's numbers in the 4th column. You will already have what the planned production was for the week, but now you will know where you ended up. With this, we see how well the production jumped when the manager knew they had to schedule more production. It is nice to see a red number move up to a yellow or green number.

By the Numbers | 69

Watch how well the office responds when the forward production target is low. You can know how well a manager is scheduling if you consistently see lower percentages. You also know that if you consistently get low percentages, and you don't make up much ground by the next week, then there may be some problems. You can also tell if your manager is a rock star if they regularly reach the production goal after starting at a low point.

Case Acceptance Rate

The case acceptance rate is one of the biggest things that most dentists don't know and don't measure. So let's measure it! The meaning of Case Acceptance Rate is how many people schedule and complete treatment when any treatment is recommended during a certain appointment. According to Dental Economics magazine in 2015, "average case acceptance is 50% to 60% for patients of record and 25% to 35% for new patients." These are troubling statistics, and they need to be improved if we are to be serving our patients and getting them the treatment they need.

> Tip: There are sometimes two ways to measure case acceptance. One is described above, and it shows on the patient level how many patients accept the treatment plan and schedule their appointment. Another way to measure this is by the dollar value. You could measure percentage of accepted treatment out of dollars of proposed treatment. When measuring, pick a methodology and keep it the same over time.

When the Doctor presents comprehensive treatment cases that are routinely above $5,000, the case acceptance is usually low. When the treatment plan is under $1,100, then case acceptance rises quite a bit, according to Kevin Rossen with Divergent Dental. This is similar to the philosophy used by Billy Beane in the book

Moneyball. Focusing on small production can move the statistics needle a lot more than trying to hit home runs all the time. Usually it's the small things like a few fillings, or just one crown. Once you start measuring the statistic, you will see if you need help in the area.

Dr. Howard Farran, owner and editor of DentalTown Magazine, always notes that most dentists are horrible at case presentation and case acceptance. He sees it as a crisis in the dental health field. He cites the statistics that it takes 3 people in your chair needing a crown, for just one person to actually receive it.

Measuring this is not easy. In simple terms, every time you finish presenting any treatment to the patient, then the staff should create a treatment plan in your practice management software. Usually it takes a practice management tracking software to track this on a large scale. After signing up for a service like this, they will walk you through how their software tracks this. If you are a multiple practice owner, this is probably the way to go because these services track in real time.

If you choose to not have a 3rd party service track this for you, there is another option. Print out two copies of every treatment plan. After a patient leaves, mark on this sheet whether they scheduled, or just left and said, "I'll look at my schedule and call you." At the end of the week, look at how many of those patients scheduled an appointment vs. how many printed plans you have with no appointment. This will give you the statistic very easily.

After seeing what your case acceptance rate is, then you can evaluate whether your front desk needs training, or whether there are systems out there that can help you make sure the patients get the care they need. Most dentists think they have high acceptance rates. More often, this is not the case, and so improving on this number can have a great impact on your practice.

> Tip: The treatment plan will include 3 items. One is how much time the doctor needs for the procedure. Let's say this is an easy filling, so we will say it will take 30 minutes, with only the central 10 minutes as captive doctor time. A "10-10-10" is how you would denote this. The second item is order in which treatment is to be done if there are multiple procedures needed. Let's say they need an extraction and then implant. In that case, you mark the extraction Level 1 importance. Then the Implant procedure gets Level 2 importance. Then Abutment and Crown get Level 3 importance. This helps the front desk staff know what stage and timing to do all appointments if the patient is to schedule right there. Then the last part will include all costs for the patient, and whether insurance will help cover any of it. The front desk staff will then be able to discuss payment methods with the patient so that they know to pay in a timely manner.

Average Online Review Score

According to Brightlocal, 90% of consumers read online reviews before visiting a business. There is also a 5 to 9% increase in revenues for each one star increase in a Yelp review according to Harvard Business Review. In this age of the internet, online reviews are not only good marketing, they are a necessity for survival and new patient flow. So how do we measure this? We will call this leading indicator the Average Online Review Score.

This statistic is a conglomeration of internet platform reviews. Online reviews give quick feedback of either positive or negative patient experiences. Many people will automatically give overall positive reviews, but a string of bad reviews might mean problems are brewing.

The three main current platforms for reviews currently are Google, Facebook, and Yelp. While many people just search Google for quality purposes, Yelp is also the platform that Apple uses in its ecosystem for information leading to both Siri and Apple Maps. Facebook is also still growing in the demographic for people ages 25-45, and so it is important to have good reviews there.

Each week, you should track how many reviews got posted online on these three platforms. If you are using any 3rd party service, then it may be automated to send out post-appointment emails asking about the entire experience. These emails then focus the positive reviews towards Google or Yelp. Hopefully each week you are adding at least 3 or more online reviews across these 3 platforms. I would also hope that they are all 5-Star reviews.

For each of these three major platforms, they all rate against a system of 1 to 5. If you got at least 3 reviews each week, then calculate the average score of the 3, or more, reviews. Put that into the tracking spreadsheet. Your goal should be to have 5-Star reviews every time.

Managing your online presence on these platforms is extremely important. Your Yelp and Google business pages must have great pictures and be monitored for any negative reviews. Your Facebook page must also have great content and pictures, as people will often look at your information across multiple platforms to check for uniformity and veracity.

It is also vitally important that you try your hardest to mitigate any negative reviews. Businesses with two negative reviews on the first page of search results are at risk of losing 44% of its customers.

Monthly LIs

NP ScRP Rate

Studies show that about 40% of the population is at risk for periodontal disease during their lifetime. Some studies have shown an even higher rate. Recent studies from cardiologists have also shown that there is a high correlation between the plaque found in coronary artery disease and periodontal pathogens. With each passing day, the research indicates that periodontal disease is a serious issue that has an effect on the entire body's health.

In the dental industry, there is rampant under-treatment of periodontitis. Many patients do not get this treatment because dentists and hygienists are afraid to confront the patient about the disease and the way that changes their treatment needs. Sometimes this is a money issue as well, since most dental insurances do not cover periodontal treatments at 100% like most 'preventative' treatments.

Although the incidence of periodontitis in the general population is around 40%, the chances that a new patient in your practice has it is closer to 60%. If a patient has gone any period of time without the proper cleanings or care, there is a good chance they have subgingival calculus and possible bone loss. Tracking this number allows you to see whether your hygienists and your dentists are potentially missing some cases of periodontitis. This number should be at or near 60%.

Similar to previous statistics, a good third party software will track this Scaling and Root Planing rate. Usually these software systems search your periodontal charts and look for high probe depths, and then see if something was missed. If you don't have this software, just go back at the end of the month and perform a chart audit yourself to see if you are hitting near the 60% of periodontitis that we know is in the population.

We all know that periodontal disease is a very tough condition to diagnose and discuss with patients. Obviously we would never want to over-treat our patients or do treatment that is not necessary. One of the best ways to feel comfortable with your diagnosis is to take your hygiene staff and yourself to some continuing education on periodontal disease. After having a few hours of CE on the disease, you and your staff can have much more informed discussions on a patient's treatment. This will lead to overall better care of your patients and save them from tooth loss in the future.

> Tip: It is also great now that the ADA has recognized the code for 'Scaling in the presence of inflammation', D4346. This is sometimes known as the 'bloody prophy'. This usually means that there is inflammation and bleeding, but no bone loss yet. This can be a great code to use when you are not quite sure whether the patient's case requires a full mouth of scaling and root planing.

Percent of Patients Referring New Patients

If you are offering high quality service and creating a good patient experience, many existing patients should refer their family and friends to you. In any practice, a certain amount of new patients should be derived from this method. Any extra marketing dollars should then bring in a stream of other patients that haven't had any friends or family meet you yet.

While this number can vary quite a bit due to geography and type of patient base, the goal should be to have 20% or more of your patient base referring in a new patient, by total volume. Once you start tracking this, you may see your numbers are higher or lower than this. Set your own goal, and track to meet that goal.

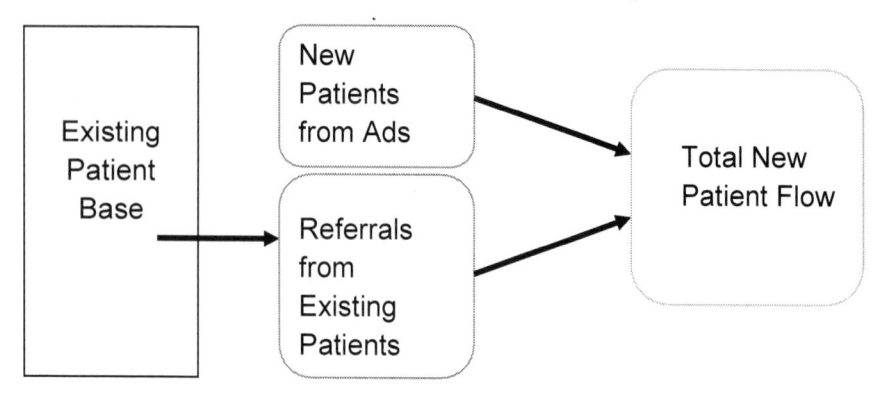

```
┌─────────────┐      ┌──────────────┐
│             │      │ New          │
│  Existing   │      │ Patients     │      ╭──────────────╮
│  Patient    │      │ from Ads     │      │              │
│  Base       │      └──────────────┘      │  Total New   │
│             │      ┌──────────────┐      │  Patient Flow│
│             │─────▶│ Referrals    │─────▶│              │
│             │      │ from         │      │              │
│             │      │ Existing     │      ╰──────────────╯
│             │      │ Patients     │
└─────────────┘      └──────────────┘
```

In the chart, it shows that you have a certain patient base that can be a referral source for you. You need to leverage this base, not only because it's free but also because it is a measure of overall practice health. If patients trust you and the clinic, they will refer their friends to you.

For example, look at a 2 doctor practice that has 5,000 patients. In a given year, they get about 70 new patients per month for the 2 doctors. That equates to 840 new patients total, of which 500 were referred by their friends, family or co-workers who already see you. So the calculation would be 500/5,000, or 10% annually. To look at this number monthly, take your total new patients referred from others, and divide it by the active patient base divided by 12. In the case above, it would be about 42 patients divided by (5,000 / 12). In this case, they need to improve that number significantly.

This is also a leading indicator for your overall patient experience. If you can provide a high level of care that exceeds expectations, then you will get many of your patients from internal referrals.

Patients will be so impressed by your office environment, your caring attitude, or the amazing patient experience, that they will send all their new co-workers your way. They may write a glowing Facebook review. Basically, this is a leading indicator as to whether you are above or below expectations in terms of the entire patient experience.

Your other source of new patients is from any marketing or advertising dollars. While marketing could technically be anything internal or external that you do to build a brand or reputation, we want to measure new patients who purely found you through other avenues. If you are tracking things well, you will be able to tell exactly which sources lead to new patients, and measure the cost per acquisition of each new patient.

For example, if you pay for postcard mailings, you will see that your budget of $500 in postcards brought in 10 patients. Usually this is tracked by patients indicating at their first visit that they found you by postcard. More savvy marketers will always put coupons on the postcard or marketing, sometimes even with trackable phone numbers or internet URL addresses. Tracking these leads is then very easy. The return on investment is then very easy to see by separating out these new patients.

You can always reward this behavior of referrals with a little something 'extra'. Sometimes this can be low-value, like a handwritten thank you card. More often, it is something that says 'Thank You' a little more. In some offices this can be a $5 or $10 gift card to a restaurant or a coffee shop. Many offices even offer a little more, as in $25 in credit to use in the office, or in a gift card to a restaurant. **In some states this is illegal**, so make sure that any system implemented stays within your state's regulations.

> Tip: Taking it a step further, you could also calculate how many different current patients are referring all these new patients to you. If only 10 people are referring 100 of new patients into your practice, that is not as good as 100 people telling one of their friends. This can be measured as the Net Promoter Score.
>
> In a survey of 1 to 10, anything 6 or below is labeled a 'Detractor'. A 7 or 8 is 'Passive', and a 9 or 10 is labeled 'Promoter'. To calculate, simply subtract the percentage of Detractors from Promoters.

The best thing about hitting this target is that it costs nothing- most of the time. If you do a great job of asking for referrals, this can often take 5 seconds, and lead to huge gains.

Tracking this takes little effort. You may have a spot in your electronic records to place this information. If you don't, make sure to write where they came from on their medical history or some other paperwork as you are meeting them for the first time. At the end of the month, go back through all new patients seen to find out how they got to your office instead of your competitor.

Re-Appointment Rate

Over 95% of your patients should be scheduled again for their next appointment. This should most often happen while the patient is still in the hygiene room, right at the end of their current hygiene appointment. This is a very easy system to put in place, as oftentimes you will allow the patient to request the best time that works for them for their next periodic exam/prophy appointment.

Tracking this most often requires using a data management software. The software can go through your database and see each day how the hygienists are doing with re-appointing every patient.

If you don't have software that can do this, then you can always add a column onto the hygiene tracking day sheet, and then keep this data written down every day until the end of the month. Usually it doesn't take long for hygienists to hit 95% as long as they know that's the goal.

If a patient chooses to leave without an appointment, it is a good idea to remind them until they get an appointment on the books. This can include phone calls once a week for a few weeks, then emails once a week for a few weeks, and then follow it up with a letter or post-card. Showing that you care about their teeth can make a huge difference and build loyalty. The quickest way to lose a patient is by indifference. If you don't care about their dental health, then they won't care about follow-up care.

> From the Data: While having a high re-appointment rate is very good, it can sometimes lead to patients booking an appointment and then not showing up for their 6 month visit. This will increase your No Show/Cancel percentage.
>
> It is imperative to have good systems to place importance on communication with the office if this future time doesn't work. It's also important to have a good confirmation and reminder system to keep the schedule full if people do change appointments on short notice.

Phone Call Close Rate

Whenever your marketing is successful, you will most likely get a lot of phone calls from new patients. When a new patient calls your office to ask for any sort of information, they are really testing your office to see if it is right for them.

Before we go any further, let's acknowledge the elephant in the room. Many phone calls to dental offices go un-answered. This is a chronic problem in dental offices where front desk employees are deluged with insurance paperwork, checking in/out patients, presenting treatment plans, collecting money, and then, if they have time, they can pick up the phone when it rings. Sometimes staff is too busy calling out to confirm appointments to answer incoming calls. Having staff ready to answer these phones is critically important to getting new patients added to the schedule! After they pick up, that's when the rubber meets the road.

It is imperative that the person answering your phone is polite, knowledgeable, and leads the prospective new patient to receiving care in your office. Sometimes we think this is easy, and it can be if your team is knowledgeable or naturally friendly. If not, training can make a key difference. The biggest reason that patients don't schedule over the phone after calling a dental office, is that staff members don't 'ask' for a patient to schedule! The simplest answer is really right in front of them the entire time, we just need to ask.

Tracking this number is almost impossible without a service like Patient Pursuit. This phone call service has human operators that listen to each phone call and grade the employee according to different metrics. When an employee is great on the phone, we will see these numbers rise and we know that our marketing dollars are truly leading to patients in the chair. If this number is low, it means that marketing leads generated are being wasted at this first point of contact. When these numbers are low, training is paramount to making sure we are not wasting money.

In some cases, all the training in the world won't help if the staff member is not made of the "right stuff". For most people, you can't change their stripes. They are either a people-person, or they're not. Finding someone who is a good people-person is a good first step to hitting this goal. A staff member with good phone skills and positive-sounding voice will convert over 85% of their phone calls.

> Tip: This percentage can be changed by many things. If your website is very informative and you have a clear marketing message, you may not get many calls that are shopping around. In these cases, most patients will call asking to schedule with a certain doctor and they have already made the decision to 'buy' what you are selling. If you have poor marketing or haphazard messaging, patients may be testing you out and price shopping. These patients would have a higher rate of no show/late cancel.

Total Patient Count

The last leading indicator of the practice is total patient count. We classify any 'active' patient as someone who has visited the office in the last 18 months. After 18 months, we can then remove the 'active' tag on them. Even though we may not get to classify them as active, it still helps to market to these patients and try to earn their business again.

Watching this number grow month to month is important because it gives you an idea on the 'back-door' of your practice. We always like to see how many new patients are coming into the office, but it's just as important to know if patients are walking out the back door of the practice. This total patient count will let us know if we are really growing the practice, or shuffling new patients in the front door as the old patients leave quietly out the back.

Days in Accounts Receivable

The Days in AR number is derived from a formula that calculates how many days, on average, it takes you to get collections for your production. This target should be under 24 days. The formula is as follows:

$$\text{Days in AR} = \frac{\text{Total Accounts Receivable}}{(\text{Sum of last 12 months total production}) / 365}$$

Here's an Example:

$$\text{Days in AR} = \frac{\$157{,}162}{\$2{,}819{,}305 / 365} = \frac{\$157{,}162}{\$7{,}724} = 20.3$$

Once you start tracking this number, you will be able to grasp the sense of how your front desk is performing, because you will see that Days in AR number fluctuate up and down. If your rock star manager leaves, you will most likely see it rise because the new replacement isn't as good at following your collections policy. Training and systemization will help keep this number low as long as all staff understand the policies you have set up.

Since the AR is usually comprised of both insurance payments in waiting and patient payments due, there are two sides that should be examined in this number. If your insurance payments are processed in a timely manner, this helps greatly. If your claim-filing process is problematic and you are getting many returned claims, then this number can rise. Submitting insurance payments electronically, and accepting electronic payments, will make a large difference in the number. Most insurance companies are trying to force providers to accept electronic payments anyway, so the industry is moving in this direction already.

If you have a large AR and lower production, you may see the Days in AR number closer to 50. In this scenario, clean up the large outstanding balances and you will see this number come back closer to your goal.

The great news is that Accounts Receivable is money that is owed to you, and all you have to do is go and get it. By instituting a tougher collections policy, you can decrease your AR to an acceptable level. Usually when an office gets strict, they will catch back up to a normal AR level within 4-6 months. During this time, all the decrease in AR comes in as 'extra' income above and beyond the normal income. This is just icing on the cake- as this is one time money - but it shows how much better it will be going forward.

Monthly KPIs

Net Monthly Production

Generally every dentist knows the provider production each week and month. This is a good number to track as a value of overall productivity. Each month, if we use our provider daily average production, we should be able to predict within a certain range what the overall production is. Knowing the production estimate, we can set goals based on this as well. Our goals can be whatever we want them to be, but these monthly production goals should always be viewed in light of our bigger goals.

Net production is the total production after you take away any in-office adjustments or outside insurance write-offs. Because write-offs tend to be recorded a month later than the production, you may see a large production month and then a wave of large write-offs in the next month.

Net production is a good thing to track over the long term, but there are factors in previous months that play a role in the upward or downward single-month swings we see.

Total production is a nice number to watch, but ultimately every time you raise your prices, the data from previous years becomes obsolete. If you raised everything across the board by 3 percent, maybe that would be a telling statistic. Rarely does that happen to such a perfect percentage level- and so that total production data can't be trusted.

Collections

Collections is what is captured of the production- "Money in the bank". We like to think that we are producing a lot of money, which should equate to a lot of collections. Unfortunately due to insurance contracts and billing practices, this isn't always the case.

Many times collections is a complicated formula which involves payments from previous work completed and prepayments for future dental work. This can also be affected by insurance payments as well as payment plans that you may have instituted within the office.

In the end, we know that our offices don't run on hopeful production numbers. They run on real cash that comes into the bank, which means collections. This number is a very important number to track so that we can pay our bills, our staff, and hopefully ourselves in the end!

Overhead Percentage

Entire books and chapters can be written on overhead percentage, but this statistic can be boiled down to the high level view. In essence, you should be tracking this total number for a while before starting to pinpoint areas where you could improve this number. After a while, you will start understanding your numbers better, and at that time you can identify the categories where you can start to save money.

Some of the later statistics in this chapter start to focus on the biggest and easiest areas of savings, but this total overhead percentage is the crucial one because it truly means what you get to take home each month.

In total, your goal for overhead percentage, excluding doctor pay, should be 60% in a general office. As you become a more well-oiled machine, and begin producing higher numbers, then your new goal should be either 55% or 50%. These very low percentages may seem like a dream that will never come true.

It is important to remember, however, that we have two categories of overhead. One is the fixed costs like rent, insurance, payments for dental software, and other expenses that are virtually always the same every month.

The other category of expenses is variable, those that go up or down with production/collections. As your production goes up, these expenses will rise. So as you increase production and become busier, your actual total dollar amount will increase. While this amount increases, the collections number increases at a faster rate, while the fixed expenses don't change. So, as your production rises, you will actually be able to achieve a lower percentage of overhead expenses and take home more of what you produce.

Collections Percent

Collections percent is the amount you collect of dollars that you are able to collect. This should typically hover around 97-99% of net production. Let's say your production is $100,000 this month, and you have $15,000 in insurance write-offs. Let's also assume that you gave $5,000 in discounts for folks who paid cash or had some sort of special discount. This means that your Net Production was $80,000 for the month. Collections percent is the total amount of money you collected out of $80,000.

It is usually best to track this number monthly, but then look at it over a 3-4 month period and average the numbers out. Due to insurance timing and when patients pay for their work, this number can fluctuate between 80% one month, and 145% the next! It is wise to not read this number too closely each month, but look at overall averages for a few months or the entire year. One tip would be to create a graph showing the collections percentage, add a trend line, and specify a 6 month moving average.

This is most often the area where many practices lose money and have the easiest time getting more of it back. Some practices have the tendency to say, "We will just send you the bill." Mrs. Jones walks out the door and thinks all is well! This truly isn't the case, and it can lead to many problems. It is wise to ask for the patient's portion the day of service, or the day when you seat/finish the procedure. In the cases where insurance may have a nebulous contract and you're not sure of the patient-responsible portion, this can be tricky.

It is then best to collect whatever you think they will end up owing. If they overpay, they will love getting a check back from you for some money. In that case, you have covered your fee and they will have a positive rush of endorphins when they see money coming back from you. In truth, they've already forgotten what they paid, and so the amount of the check can usually be quite small, but still produce the same pleasant surprise. Be sure to cut refund checks as soon as the overpayment is verified.

In the case where the patient will still owe money after insurance, then you can ask them for that payment. Remember that every time you have to chase a patient for money, it costs you money in employee time, mailing costs and costs of the materials you've already purchased and used, without any reimbursement. Think of it as a loan from yourself to yourself, but without earning any interest. Quite the opposite; it is costing you money. Therefore, it is important to try to get a very accurate assessment of insurance payments in order to have the patient pay their portion the same day treatment is performed.

> From the Data: Divergent Dental recently ran a report across hundreds of practices and found a significant correlation. Practices averaging over $200,000 in collections are averaging 101% collection percentage. Practices collecting $50,000-$200,000 are averaging 98.3% collections. Those practices collecting under $50,000 are averaging 87.4% collections.

New Patients/Month

Ask a group of dentists for the ideal number of new patients per month and you will hear numbers across a wide range, but a reasonable number per doctor is 25 per month. It is wise to track this number, because this really tells you how your internal and external marketing efforts are paying off. Internally, if you have a great patient experience with amazing customer service, you will get new patients immediately just from word of mouth. This way, you don't have to spend a single dollar on marketing and you can drive very high numbers of new patients to your practice.

External marketing can also be measured by this statistic. If you spend a lot of money on either post cards, websites, or any external marketing, you want to see the return-on-investment for that money you're spending. This is seen in how many new patients are being driven via each marketing dollar you are spending. In the new patient numbers, it is always a good idea to track how they heard about you. Hopefully it's the 'free' method of internal referrals, but if not, we want to know if our marketing dollars were spent well. Maybe they will say they saw a billboard, or maybe a postcard.

In all, 25 new patients a month per doctor is quite a bit, more than 1 new patient per working day if the doctor is working 4 to 5 days a week. A new patient is always more likely to have work that may be needed, so new patients are very important to a successful and profitable practice. Watching this number is a very important statistic because it will make a difference in how you use marketing dollars and whether you continue to invest in some of the marketing methods you've used in the past.

Doctor Production as a Percent of Total Production

Typically a practice will have 75% of production from the doctor's schedule. In a given hour, a doctor can produce much higher dollar volumes than any hygiene department because of the complexity and skill required to do things like crowns, implants, and endodontics. Generally this leads to about a 75%-25% split between the doctor and hygiene.

If you start to see a higher doctor production percentage, it might mean that hygiene is under-producing. This could mean they aren't doing enough periodontal procedures, or maybe not offering enough adjunct services. As a high quality doctor, you probably have a standard of care that you would want for your family or best friends. If your hygiene department isn't living up to those standards, they may not be pulling in the production that they should.

However, it may also be the case that you as the doctor are functioning at a very high level. This could mean that you do many high dollar procedures or work very diligently. If this is the case, then a higher percentage is understandable. However, if you are killing yourself to get through 20 patients a day doing a lot of dentistry, you risk burn-out. Watch this statistic to make sure that you are not working at a level that you can't sustain for a considerable amount of time. If you are working too hard, and seeing that *'Number of Days to Next Doctor Rock Appointment'* increase, then maybe it is time to consider raising fees, ending participation with poor- paying insurance plans, or adding an associate doctor.

If the hygiene production percentage is too high vs. the doctor production percentage, it could mean a few things. First, it could mean that the doctor has a very large hygiene base that is in regular recalls. This large base of patients in the recall cycle may not need much work, but having 3 hygienists working the schedule creates quite a bit of production. This scenario would be acceptable. The other possibility is that the doctor is under-producing for what is typical. This may mean the doctor is referring out too many procedures that could be kept in-house, or potentially not treatment-planning to a typical standard of care. This can be hard to see sometimes, but watching this number over time may tell you if of these things are happening in your practice.

Insurance Write-Off Percentage

In today's competitive marketplace, joining insurance Preferred Provider Organizations (PPOs) is sometimes necessary to build up a patient base and become a viable business. Insurance companies have greatly increased the access to care by broadening the possible patients who see their routine dental care as "free." While we all know it's not "free," patients feel like it's something their employer offers and it is often free to their after-tax dollars.

Now that we've identified some of the positives of insurance, there are a few negatives. With the explosion of dental insurance companies in the marketplace, there are some plans that are very restrictive in benefits and may pay at an extremely low rate. This can be positively depressing if you join one of these plans and they pay at a very low reimbursement rate. Some of these plans pay at such a low percentage that it may seem like you are losing money on each procedure. This may actually be the case, but to know for sure, you will need to do a little homework.

Your first step is to perform a cost analysis. You need to determine what it costs you to do almost every procedure in your practice. For example, add up the cost of the 2 pieces of gauze, the length of floss, the matrix band and everything else associated with a one-surface filling. In this formula, you will also need to figure out what it takes to open your office for 1 hour and have a chair available for one hour. This cost will include wages, benefits and payroll taxes for front office and clinical staff, electricity, rent and any other costs associated with just opening the doors for that one hour. Then take those costs and look at what you get paid by each insurance company. If an insurance company isn't covering the procedure and profit margin, you may decide that you should not participate with that plan. This process is done in more detailed in the section 'Numbers to Track Intermittently.'

Overall, watching this insurance write-off percentage will be important whenever you want to start seeing if you can increase collections. By going 'Out of Network' with some of these PPOs, you can see your insurance write-off percentage drop, and hopefully increase your take home collections. This can often cause patients to leave your practice, but the positive financial impact can be greater than the loss of patients. This also opens up availability with the doctor and hygienists for people who will be paying more for those services.

Lab Percentage of Overhead

One of the biggest cost categories that is easy for general dentists to manage is the laboratory percentage. If you are doing a lot of lab work, that means you are probably doing some good high-production dentistry. This can be great for your production and collections numbers, but it also does increase the bill that you will owe some lab technicians in the following month. Typically we like to see this category around 6%.

To hit that percentage, you will need to maximize a few things. First, you will need to evaluate the lab market and see what your costs are in comparison to the general marketplace. Remember, "Knowledge is power." With this knowledge, you then have the power to decide whether you want to keep your current lab or perhaps try out other labs that have lower fees. This can sometimes be difficult if you have a great relationship with a lab, but what if keeping your lab tech meant a decrease in your retirement account of $250,000?

If you like your current lab, maybe they will be willing to match the prices you see from other labs. This would be great, as then they keep your business and you get to save money instantly. If not, then start trying out other labs to see if they can produce similarly high quality crowns, bridges and dentures for less.

One thing to watch out for is sending lab work overseas or to labs that may use materials that come from non-satisfactory sources. There has been a boom in Zirconia manufactured in China that doesn't conform to the same standards as the name brand Zirconia crowns. Make sure your labs prove to you that they are using Zirconia made to the finest standards.

With some negotiations, you should be able to get down to the 6% mark. Some months, it may not be possible to get down to that level, but that means that you were doing lots of high-production dentistry, and that is also good for the overall health of the business.

Supply Percentage of Overhead

The next important part of your overhead is dental supplies. This can be similarly tough to get down, because we all have our favorite matrix or impression materials that we like to use. The great advantage we currently have is the ability to search the internet for better prices, and leverage that knowledge to get better rates from suppliers. Typically an office will run around 6-8% for dental supplies, but the goal should be to target it at 4%.

The first step to control these costs is to come up with a supply *formulary*. This is the entire list of every single item you have ordered or plan on ordering in the next few months. There will always be items that you only order once in a lifetime, like some new instruments, and we can take that off this list. This list will be a comprehensive list of everything you will need to run the office and on which any staff member could just check a box to order a certain number of units.

For this exercise, let's create a spreadsheet. Every supply item you will order is in column A, and vendors are in subsequent columns. The vendors could be the big players, mail catalogs, or small online vendors. In each of these columns, put the price you would be charged for these items. Maybe they offer a generic brand of the product- and that price could be added in as well. Make sure that any shipping costs are added in if charged by the item.

After you come up with this list, you will see the cost savings you could achieve by switching some of your ordering from one company to one or more different companies. This takes a lot of initial work, but the cost savings year over year can be significant and rewarding.

Sometimes savings come from ordering generic versions of a product, and sometimes the fees are different from one warehouse to another. This savings can be upwards of 50% on some products. As the news has reported in recent years, there is a growing gray market on products that are manufactured internationally and then shipped to the US for higher price sales. With this gray market, always be wary of using products like composite, bonding, and other materials that are volatile under heat or deteriorate over time. You want to use quality materials, don't you? The good news is that many products such as sterilization materials, plastic trays, patient napkins, and other paper products aren't affected by heat or time.

Once you've come to the realization that you can save lots of money with supplies, the goal is to hit that target every month. Most likely, the doctor is not the one submitting the order every week. It is probably an assistant or hygienist. The best way to manage this expense category is to meet with this person and explain to them the total budget for the month. If they keep track of their order totals every week, then they will know when they start getting close to the budgeted amount for the month. If they have to submit an order over that budget amount, then they will need to get approval from the doctor before submitting that order. After a few months of this system, the ordering person will be able to hold this cost category in check. A typical savings amount would be 2-3% of revenue. With an average practice collecting $600,000, this can save you $12,000-$18,000 a year.

Now that we've explained how you would do it the hard way, we can now talk about how technology has changed the game. Recently there's been much progress in the online ordering business and vendors are encouraged to plainly state their price and give fair fees to both large groups and single-doctor offices. This has started to level the playing field and has allowed everyone to get better prices.

Some of these websites are very good, but sometimes the best ones require fees. On the website addisonkilleen.com, look under 'Resources' and find today's most recommended system. There are even programs these days that automate all aspects of the supply budget, recommend possible generic replacements, and initiate order tracking so that it saves your staff time and energy.

Staff Payroll Percentage of Overhead

The largest single category of the overhead is the staff costs. Staff costs include front desk, insurance coordinator, and dental assistant wages, benefits, and payroll taxes. (Hygiene payroll will be dealt with in the next section.) This can be a touchy subject for some dentists who are close to their staff, and it is one that is not very fun to talk about. The target percentage is 16%. I'm not recommending that you go out immediately and reduce any employee wages until the total hits the target, because this can sometimes cause a staff revolt and you can experience some work-flow issues resulting from mass-exodus.

Setting staff wages accordingly can be tough if you're in a tight labor market or in a rural area where you are competing for a finite resource. However, it is wise to track this number to pay at the market rate, and not above it just because the employee has gone around the sun a few more times.

Setting appropriate wages is a complicated but worthwhile use of time. Using length of time served inside your organization is a good baseline, but the appropriate wage should focus more on skills and production by that employee. If that employee is fantastic at CAD/CAM crown designing or Invisalign©, you might increase their wage due to these skills.

I also don't recommend lowering anyone's wages to hit this mark. This can be a very negative tone to set in the office and can lead to a lot of staff turnover. This turnover can be even costlier as you have to train more employees in a new system. It is usually better to track this number over the long term and evaluate all business decisions knowing where this category is. As you increase production, your percentage in staffing costs will decrease down to a better level.

> Note: It is widely proven by studies and research that employees want an encouraging, happy work environment more than a raise. Sometimes this can include small financial tokens, but doesn't necessarily have to mean long-term increases in wage. One method that can be very useful is a random gift card given to an employee who has been demonstrating especially good characteristics.

Hygiene Payroll Percentage of Overhead

Another large part of staffing costs that we excluded from the last statistic was hygiene payroll. This is usually targeted at 9% of revenues. Remember that the target hygiene percentage of total production is 25%. This 9% is about ⅓ of that production, which is ideal. Typically a hygienist will make ⅓ of their collections in their department. Now there are many different ways to go about deciding what is 'hygiene collections', but I have no opinion as to whether that includes retail sales of toothbrushes or other adjunct products. The only guidance I will give is that you must track numbers the same way over time in order to know how those numbers change.

The same guidance given in the last section about staff costs applies here. It is not wise to reset your hygiene wages in order to hit this goal. A better move would be to educate your hygienists up to the level where they will be producing closer to a market rate. Investing in good CE can make a huge difference in knowledge and treatment of periodontal disease. In the same fashion, if you prefer to use a certain type of toothbrush at home, why not offer that same toothbrush to patients to purchase in your office? Many times, a toothbrush company will sell to you at a discount rate, and you can save patients money if you sell it in the office. A few strategies like this will help you get closer to this 9% target number.

Production per Chair

This is a metric that is good to measure over time to track trends. As I stated in the beginning of the book, each metric must have a useful action plan if there are trends in the number. This metric is no different.

To calculate this number, take net production divided by the number of patient operatories you have in the practice.

If you see this number increase, then it may be time for an extra chair. Adding that extra chair can mean that you may be able to increase production by another multiple of a chair if you add it.

There will certainly be a lag, and this new chair may require more staff costs, but revenues could increase while keeping most fixed costs, excluding staff, at the same level.

Daily Production per Provider

This is a great statistic to track over time because it can lead to many insights. Specifically we want to track each individual provider-- hygienists as well as dentists. To arrive at a daily figure, find the monthly production for the provider, and then divide by how any days they worked. By this method, you avoid comparing production from a month with only 17 working days with production from a month with 22 working days.

For hygienists, it can be useful to see if some employees are working harder than others. Sometimes you will see long-term trends in terms of dollars produced per hour. Trends could have different causes. In one scenario, one hygienist could be working harder than another, and seeing more patients in that day. However, that hygienist could also be going too fast for good patient care. In that case, they may not be doing everything you expect of a hygienist, and not helping out in other areas of the practice, such as sterilization. In turn, if a hygienist is a consistently low producer, it could be that they aren't offering procedures that you would prefer they do. This could include treatments like fluoride varnish, sealants, and scaling and root planing. The addition of these little treatments can alleviate some of the backlog in the doctor's schedule, and also create more revenue in the hygiene department. One way to check on the uniformity of production is to have a checklist for hygiene, where each appointment has to go through each step. The cause of any discrepancies will be found once you evaluate to make sure these checklists are being completed.

For dentists, daily production can vary a lot month to month. That is completely understandable if you have some months where you do a lot of expensive dentistry, and others where you are doing fillings all day long. However, your production numbers should fall into a consistent range. If you do more expensive procedures like implants, endodontics, and orthodontics, your daily numbers can be much higher than if you are doing fillings and dentures. Over time, track this number and see how the trends are affected by changes that you can make.

For dentists, continuing education on some of the more complicated procedures can lead to increased daily production levels. Things like molar root canals and implants can have huge effects on production. Over time, if you enjoy doing these procedures, then you will see an increase in your daily production average.

This number also helps predict what the monthly income is going to be in the future. After you figure out what the doctor production is, then add up how many hygienists will be working each day, and then you will arrive at the daily production numbers for each month. Going forward, you can use this number to budget and see, with pretty good accuracy, what your clinic's monthly production will be.

Here is the summarized Scorecard that you should be able to review at the end of each month. To track these numbers every month, go to my website, addisonkilleen.com, and download a copy.

Leading Indicators LI		Key Production Indicators KPI	
Weekly		**Monthly**	
# of days to next NP	<7 days	Net Production	
# of days to next Rock appointment	<7 days	Collections	
Fluoride Rate	>90%	Overhead% (Exc-Dr)	<60%
CX/NS	<4 %	Collections %	>99% Ave.
Forward Production target	(Sheet)	New Patients/month	>25/Doc
Case Acceptance Rate	>90%	Doc% of Total Production	75%
Ave. Online Review Score	5	Ins Write-off %	
Monthly		Lab %	6%
NP ScRP Rate	>40%	Supply %	4%
% of Patients referring NP	>20%	Staff Payroll %	16%
Days in AR	< 24 Days	Hyg. Payroll %	9%
Re-Appoint Rate	>95%	Production/Chair	
Phone Call Close Rate	>85%	Daily Prod per Provider	
Total Patient Count	Increasing		

Numbers to Track Intermittently

Cost per Procedure

Whether we are doing a one-surface filling, or a buildup and crown, dentists usually don't know the cost of production. This flies in the face of almost every principle of business known in the world. How much can you sell that machine for if you don't know what it cost to build it? How much can you sell that sandwich for if you don't know the cost of its ingredients? You get the picture. Costs per procedure can be very easy to figure out-- and here are the steps:

1. Fixed Costs per Month: This will include rent, utilities, tech costs, any contracted services you purchase, staffing costs (excluding doctor pay), insurance costs, and any other services that usually stay about the same each month. You will probably get a large number, and then divide that number by the number of hours the office is seeing patients, on average, per month. If you normally work 4.5 days a week, then maybe that is about 18 days per month at an 8 hour day, so about 144 hours. Once you come down to an hourly fixed cost- then you need to divide by the number of chairs you have actively available in the office. Sometimes this number will be $10/chair/hour, sometimes it is $25/chair/hour. This is the first number to plug in. Place that at the top of the spreadsheet. Multiply this number by the number of hours this chair will be used start-to-finish for this specific procedure.
2. Quantities of all supplies for that procedure: In any procedure, you may want to go through, step-by-step, with your assistant to see exactly how much of each item is used. This will need to be identified down to number

of Q-tips, pieces of 2x2 gauze, length of floss, amount of PVS impression material, etc. Once you identify the quantity of each supply, place that in a spreadsheet with the name and quantity. Don't forget sterilization costs for the procedure as well, including number of bags used afterwards, and possibly number of Cavi-wipes.
3. Cost of supplies: Once you have each supply that goes into a procedure, you need to find out the cost for each. If there are 2000 gauze 2x2s in a box for $24, then you need to divide that cost and arrive at the cost of 1.2 cents per gauze. Do this for each supply, and you will come up with the total supply cost for the procedure.
4. Lab Costs: This one is easy to figure out. If it is crown or bridge, you just add the unit price onto the bottom. If it's dentures, add that cost.

In the end you will arrive at the total cost per procedure. This is a very useful number for two reasons. First, you can use this number to evaluate insurance or discount plans. If it costs $140 to do a crown in total, and you're getting $350 from a particular insurance plan, then it may be to your benefit to accept that plan. However, if you are only getting $225 to do it, and the doctor is potentially taking 30% of production as pay, then it probably is too tight a margin to make it worthwhile.

You can also use this number to evaluate scheduling. If your profit margins are thin on some procedures, then you need to see how many hours of chair-time they are taking. If a particular procedure takes too long, then the hourly chair cost goes up, and could potentially impact the profitability of that procedure. If that were the case, then you could always schedule something else in another chair to make sure the office was making money that hour rather than experiencing a possible loss.

New Patient Income

Income per new patient is good to measure because new patients often make up the bulk of the profitability in a mature office. Usually the revenues from new patients are higher than from existing patients, because they will likely have a problem that is bringing them in, have more severe periodontal situations, or have neglected their teeth for a period of time.

This metric is calculated by taking the total number of new patients during a 6 month time period divided by the income from treatment of those patients during that same time period. This number can lead to a more accurate assessment of the value of marketing dollars when trying to acquire new patients. If it costs $100 to get that patient in the door, but you have revenues of $1,000 on them, then you most likely have covered your costs and made some profit during that first 6 months. After that, you know you have paid for the marketing dollars and hopefully you can keep that patient for life if you maintain a high quality of care.

Patient Value

This number is a good metric to determine the value each patient has to the practice each year. To arrive at this number, you take the total patient number divided by the total revenues of the practice over that same time frame. Notice we are talking about people seen, not appointments kept. So if there were 2000 patients seen in that year, and revenues were $761,100, then the resulting patient value would be $380/patient over that year.

> Note: Active Patients is defined as the number of patients seen over the last 18 months. If it has been 18 months + 1 day, then it is assumed they have left the practice- or are no longer part of your practice for statistical purposes.

This can be a great tool to use in budgeting and future forecasting. If you know that your patient base is growing, it will usually give you a somewhat reliable forecast as to what revenues will be for the future. This can also be used to justify what kind of marketing efforts you are using, and the costs. If you are spending $100/patient to get them in the door, then you know the profitability of your investment as long as the patient decides to stay with your practice.

Procedure Mix

This evaluation centers on the types of procedures that a doctor is completing, and the financial impact that has on their production. To complete this evaluation, simply run a report of all procedures done over a certain period of time, and then also include the total production amount associated with these procedures. It is best to run this report using data for 3 months or longer, because one month's statistics can show abnormal spikes in some areas.

Export all the "D####" codes and production associated with them. Using a spreadsheet you can then isolate out which category each procedure falls into, and then carry over the dollar amount of production associated with that procedure. The resulting totals from each section should be able to create a nice pie chart of the procedure mix that each doctor is doing, weighted by production amount.

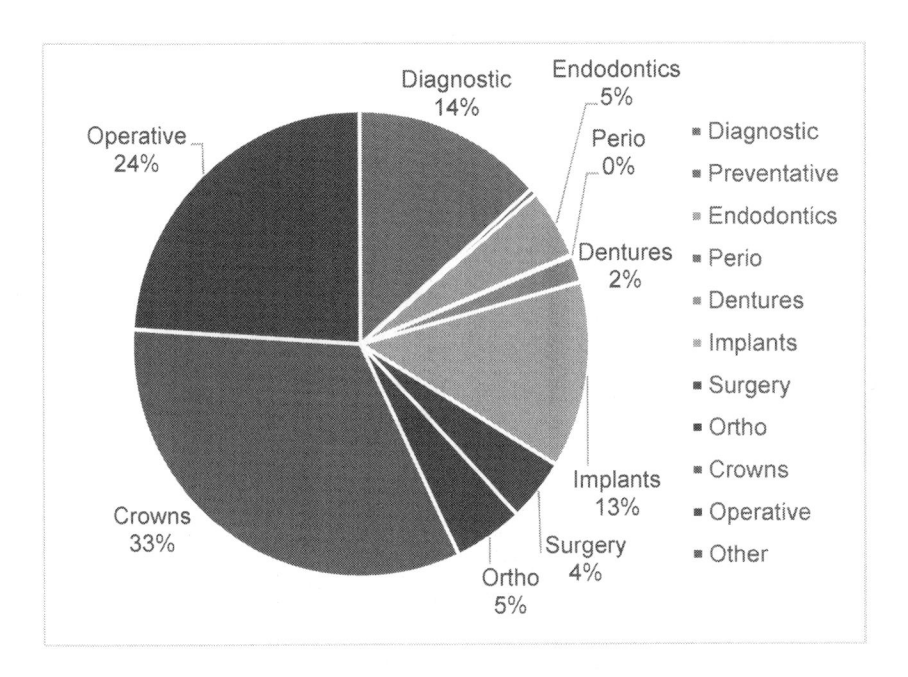

Pie chart showing procedure distribution: Diagnostic 14%, Endodontics 5%, Perio 0%, Dentures 2%, Implants 13%, Surgery 4%, Ortho 5%, Crowns 33%, Operative 24%. Legend: Diagnostic, Preventative, Endodontics, Perio, Dentures, Implants, Surgery, Ortho, Crowns, Operative, Other.

The pie chart is good when looking at one doctor, but if you have multiple doctors, you can also put them into stacked bar graphs. The overall height of the bars shows total production, and can be used to compare doctors if they work similar hours or days per month.

This exercise is particularly valuable in a couple of circumstances. The first would be when evaluating a potential practice purchase. If you want to validate what procedures a selling doctor is completing, this is very useful. Sometimes a doctor may say they do a lot of endodontics, but the numbers will not lie. Using this also lets a purchasing doctor know if there are any potential areas for growth after the practice purchase. If a selling doctor doesn't do any endodontics, you should be able to surmise that you can increase that percentage and thereby increase income by a certain amount.

By the Numbers | 105

All Doctors Chart

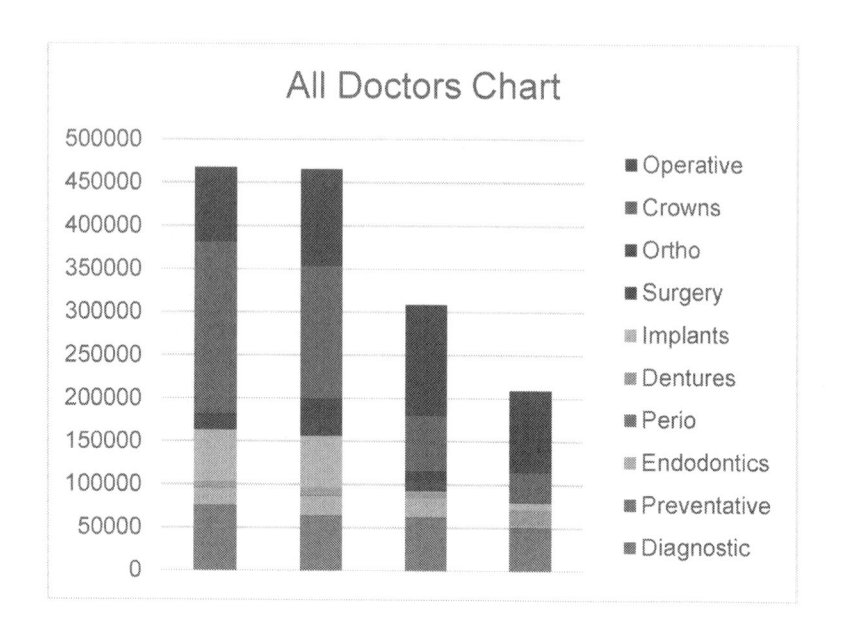

Stacked bar chart showing four doctors with procedure categories: Operative, Crowns, Ortho, Surgery, Implants, Dentures, Perio, Endodontics, Preventative, Diagnostic. Y-axis ranges from 0 to 500000.

The other potential use for this exercise is to evaluate associate doctors in a group setting. With multiple doctors, you can then compare what a senior doctor is doing versus a new associate who may not be comfortable with everything. Senior doctors should be considered the 'gold standard' when it comes to procedure mix as well as clinical standards in general. Using these doctors as the measuring tool, it is then easy to coach an associate doctor in what areas they can grow to be more successful as an all-around doctor.

> Note: It isn't always the doctor's skill set that dictates the procedure mix. The location and demographics may dictate the overall procedure mix. If a practice is in a low socioeconomic area, or high in Medicaid population, this may lead to more extractions and dentures. Whereas, if a practice is in the suburbs in a high-end shopping area, the practice may do more cosmetic veneers, crowns, and implants.

Final Notes

The amount of information created in the world in a given day is staggering- almost 2.5 billion gigabytes of data per day. There are tons of content being pushed out in every corner of the world concerning business, dentistry and every other subject under the sun. Some platforms try to piggy-back on our evolutionary dopamine reward system, as they try to feed large amounts of data into our simple brains. This has a reverse effect on the understanding of the data. If we try to understand all these data points, we will surely fail. The keys are to find the 'actionable intelligence' and act on those few data points.

Thankfully, you will not need to know everything about business to be a fantastic business owner and to be wildly successful. To be successful, however, you will need to focus on a few things that make the most difference. It's like Pareto's Rule- also known as the 80-20 rule: 80% of the results come from 20% of the effort. Focus on the small number of statistics in this book and you will be able to take your dental practice to amazing heights!

As I've mentioned throughout the chapters, check out the website (addisonkilleen.com) to find some of the resources needed to execute this system. These spreadsheets and documents will help you open your eyes to the most important data.

If you have any questions after reading this book, please don't hesitate to reach out to me by email on my website. I check my email daily (yes, I know that's an unproductive habit), and will try to email back with any help as needed. I am also found on the Dental Success Network (dentalsuccessnetwork.com). Thank you for reading this book and I hope you enjoyed the information!

Made in the USA
Lexington, KY
19 June 2018